Substance Use, End-of-Life Care and Multiple Deprivation

Focussing on end-of-life care for people who use, or have used, substances, this book explores their social and health care needs and the multiple disadvantages they have often experienced, discussing the complexities around access to care that result.

Presenting models of good practice, case studies and empirically based evidence, *Substance Use and End-of-Life Care and Multiple Deprivation* is informative, rigorous and useful for policy and practice development. The first section foregrounds the personal experiences of people living with substance use, their families and friends, and the health and social care professionals who work with them. The second section looks at how health inequalities can impact people in need of palliative care, including chapters on health literacy, mental health and learning disabilities. The final section explores social challenges that may be experienced, including homelessness, sex work, racism and incarceration.

This interdisciplinary volume is essential for researchers, practitioners, students and educators working around substance use, mental health and palliative and end-of-life care, who are looking for guidance and a reference for their work in supporting people at the end of their lives who have multiple and often complex needs.

Gary Witham is a Senior Lecturer in Nursing at Manchester Metropolitan University, UK. His research interests are exploring marginalised populations' experiences and access to palliative and end-of-life care services. Specifically, he has co-investigated the experiences of people using substances at the end of life, their carers and family as well as health and social care professionals. He has also worked on projects exploring the implementation of good practice models of care related to support people using substances at the end of life.

Sarah Galvani is Professor of Substance Use and Social Research at Manchester Metropolitan University, UK. Sarah is a social worker by profession, having started out working as a volunteer in the UK and USA with homeless people with mental ill health and/or people who use alcohol or other drugs. As an academic, she currently leads work on end-of-life and palliative care for people using substances and focusses on substance-related research among marginalised populations.

Sam Wright joined Professor Sarah Galvani and a multi-disciplinary team at Manchester Metropolitan University in 2016 to work on a large exploratory study focussing on end-of-life care for people with alcohol and other drug problems. Her main focus has been interviewing people approaching the end of life, their family caregivers and the health practitioners working with them. More recently she has been helping to develop a new model of end-of-life care for people using substances in Liverpool and Sefton (UK) and also evaluating effective ways of supporting people who are street homeless.

Gemma A. Yarwood is a Senior Lecturer in Criminology and Sociology, Manchester Metropolitan University, UK. A key focus of Gemma's research is end-of-life care and substance use. Her research informs the core curriculum of the top 10 rated MA/MSc/BA/BSc Criminology and Sociology degrees which she delivers at Manchester Metropolitan University. She has written for many publications, including journal articles, website content, book chapters, reports for various organisations and national charities.

Routledge Research in Nursing and Midwifery

For more information about this series, please visit: https://www.routledge.com/Routledge-Research-in-Nursing/book-series/RRIN

Substance Use, End-of-Life Care and Multiple Deprivation

Practice and Research

Edited by
Gary Witham, Sarah Galvani,
Sam Wright and Gemma A. Yarwood

Routledge
Taylor & Francis Group

LONDON AND NEW YORK

First published 2023
by Routledge
4 Park Square, Milton Park, Abingdon, Oxon OX14 4RN

and by Routledge
605 Third Avenue, New York, NY 10158

Routledge is an imprint of the Taylor & Francis Group, an informa business

British Library Cataloguing-in-Publication Data
A catalogue record for this book is available from the British Library

Library of Congress Cataloging-in-Publication Data
Names: Witham, Gary, editor. | Galvani, Sarah, editor. | Yarwood, Gemma A. (Gemma Anne), editor.
Title: Substance use, end of life care and multiple deprivation : practice and research / edited by Gary Witham, Sarah Galvani, Gemma A. Yarwood.
Other titles: Routledge research in nursing and midwifery.
Description: Abingdon, Oxon ; New York, NY : Routledge, 2023. | Series: Routledge research in nursing and midwifery | Includes bibliographical references and index. |
Identifiers: LCCN 2022025170 (print) | LCCN 2022025171 (ebook) | ISBN 9781032035468 (hardback) | ISBN 9781032372921 (paperback) | ISBN 9781003187882 (ebook)
Subjects: MESH: Substance-Related Disorders—therapy | Terminally Ill | Terminal Care—methods | Palliative Care—methods | Drug Users—psychology | Social Deprivation | United Kingdom
Classification: LCC RC564 (print) | LCC RC564 (ebook) | NLM WM 270 | DDC 616.86029—dc23/eng/20220727
LC record available at https://lccn.loc.gov/2022025170
LC ebook record available at https://lccn.loc.gov/2022025171

ISBN: 978-1-032-03546-8 (hbk)
ISBN: 978-1-032-37292-1 (pbk)
ISBN: 978-1-003-18788-2 (ebk)

DOI: 10.4324/9781003187882

Typeset in Goudy
by codeMantra

Dedication

For Maddy, Zak and Teddy, for teaching me about love, beauty and strength (GW).

For my wonderful Uncle, Dave Evans, who filled my childhood with happy memories, my adolescence with love and laughter, and my adulthood with warmth, support and pride (SG).

For my dad, Bob Wright, from whom I inherited my gentle curiosity about people and my quiet subversiveness (SW).

For Mark Brookfield, who didn't quite make the year and my co-editors who supported me with generous hearts. In the darkest moments friends shine light. (GY).

Contents

Figures

Tables

Boxes

Contributors

Anya Ahmed is Professor of Wellbeing and Communities at Manchester Metropolitan University. As a social scientist, Anya's research has explored the social aspects of ageing, migration, housing, homelessness and dementia with a focus on the experiences of Black and minoritised communities. Professor Ahmed's academic background is in social policy and social justice, exploring social inequalities among for older people from marginalised communities, who are frequently absent from the narrative on ageing and from research generally.

Jo Ashby is Head of the Department of Psychology at Manchester Metropolitan University. Jo's interests lie within the field of social and health psychology with a specific interest in substance misuse and community treatment, particularly alcohol misuse, and how treatment programmes have the potential to bring about positive behaviour change long-term. Jo was the lead qualitative researcher for a wider funded project led by Professor Sarah Galvani that aimed to explore the experiences of end–of-life care for substance misusers. More recently Jo is working on projects that aim to explore identities of behaviour change for people in long-term recovery.

Adele Brien is a Clinical Nurse Specialist in Palliative Care working in an inner city area of Manchester, UK. She holds a BSc Hons in Nursing and is an Independent Nurse Prescriber and works as part of a multidisciplinary team. Adele is passionate about working in the community setting caring for patients and their families in their own home and ensuring they are represented and have access to all services. She welcomes the challenges of palliative patients with substance misuse issues and ensuring their needs are met while approaching end of life.

Niamh Brophy has worked in the field of homelessness and palliative care for the last seven years. She has recently set up a homeless palliative care service for St Ann's hospice, working across Greater Manchester. Niamh previously held a similar role at St Mungo's in London, working to ensure individuals receive care that best meets their medical, nursing, psychological, social and spiritual needs so they can approach the end of their life with dignity and respect, and ensures the homeless sector staff working with them are also supported. Niamh also works as an integrative therapist with a special interest in trauma, and its impact on recovery and wellbeing.

Lorna Chesterton is a researcher at Manchester Metropolitan University specialising in social ageing and dementia within marginalised groups. Her research interests centre on how people's culture, ethnicity, beliefs and socio-economic situations impact upon their health and access to services. Lorna's work is grounded in a person-centred approach to research and care, valuing the contribution which individuals' personal experience can make to research and future service provision. This book chapter has allowed us to highlight some of the challenges facing Black and minoritised communities' access to services for palliative care, and substance use.

Amanda Clayson has a personal investment in recovery-based research. She is exploring her own 'recovery journey' (alcohol and eating disorders) and working closely with others to explore theirs. She is a trained teacher, Registered General Nurse and a Learning Disability Nurse. She is the founder of VoiceBox Inc., an organisation grounded firmly in community networks, explicitly aimed at enhancing the influence and impact of lived experience across community, practice and policy arenas. Her work around end-of-life care continues to help open up this often hidden area for people touched by substance use. She is a long-term Community Research Partner with Manchester Metropolitan University.

Alison Colclough retired in December 2021 following 35 years as a qualified nurse. She finished her career as St. Luke's (Cheshire) Hospice Palliative Homelessness Service Lead. She has ten plus years' experience of working voluntarily at a Homelessness shelter where she noted the real inequalities for those with no fixed address and those using substances. In 2013 St. Luke's asked her to establish a dedicated service for those experiencing homelessness. This has grown and flourished into a service which now covers 3 hospices and the whole of Cheshire.

Cherilyn Dance currently works as a researcher on a freelance basis having retired from full-time employment. She has previously worked at King's College, London, the University of Bedfordshire and Manchester Metropolitan University on a variety of research projects related to children's and adults' social care. Studies that she has worked on that are particularly relevant in the context of this volume include a major study focussed on social workers' experiences of working with problematic alcohol or drug use and she was part of a team headed by Prof Sarah Galvani which examined end-of-life care for people who have substance use issues.

Peter Higgs is a Burnet Senior Fellow and the co-head of the alcohol and other drugs working group. He has over 25 years' experience working in teaming, research and community development both in Australia and overseas. Dr Higgs works with marginalised populations in the areas of drug use and blood-borne virus treatment, prevention and transmission. His work is published widely and has included documenting the dynamic nature of street-based heroin markets across Melbourne highlighting the potential health problems for street-based injecting drug users and the evolving transmission of blood-borne viruses in active injectors.

Marian Peacock is a Senior Lecturer in Public Health at Edge Hill University and Honorary Lecturer in Public Health at the University of Sheffield. Her teaching and research interests are in developing and extending sociological perspectives on health inequalities and the place of neoliberalism in sharpening inequality and its health consequences. In recent years she has worked on a range of research projects including the Both Sides of the Fence study on improving end-of-life care for prisoners.

Mary Turner is a Reader in Health Services Research at the University of Huddersfield. She is a qualified nurse and had a lengthy career in oncology and palliative care nursing, in both clinical practice and leadership roles, before completing her PhD at King's College London and moving into a research career. Her recent work includes research into advance care planning during COVID-19 and integrated care for older people approaching the end of life in the community. She has a particular interest in ageing and dying in prison, and she is currently leading an international task force on palliative care for prisoners for the European Association for Palliative Care (EAPC).

Lucy Webb is a Reader in psychosocial health at Manchester Metropolitan University, UK. Her academic interests in psychosocial health developed when studying psychology, attaining a Masters and then a PhD in health psychology. She is also a member of the Society for the Study of Addiction. Lucy established the Co-production in Addiction Network for the Collaborative Centre for Values-Based Practice, at St. Catherine's College, Oxford, and her recent work incorporates co-production and participatory methodologies to maximise representation and social inclusion. She is currently involved in researching end-of-life care for people with problematic substance use.

Foreword

Palliative care has come a long way since its beginnings as a hospice movement in 1960s England. Before that time, aggressive and unnecessary treatments prevailed for people with life-limiting illnesses. Poor symptom management and ideas about medical secrecy and medical failure led to institutional embarrassment and patient disenfranchisement and stigma. The last 20 years have witnessed palliative care become beneficial and benevolent features of health care systems around the world. Symptom management and access, especially for cancer patients in affluent countries, has vastly improved. However, access and quality of care beyond these privileged groups remain a serious and continuing challenge.

This book brings together a collection of writers and researchers to showcase the significant inequities and inequalities in palliative care for people living in circumstances of deprivation – poverty, homelessness, welfare and in lifestyles characterised by long-term substance use. These populations often hold intersectional factors that compound their inequality – geographical, gendered, racial and sexual inequality, as well as intellectual or developmental disability. The plight of these social and cultural populations in our modern societies highlight how much more urgently needs to be done in end-of-life care. For these people, policy invisibility, stigma and marginalisation by professional actions, and omission of strategies to address these deficits and prejudices all represent a glaring social injustice in our midst.

By moving from a solely clinical approach to palliative care to one that adopts a social model of care we can begin to address this social justice dimension of caring in a compassionate and inclusive way. This kind of public health approach to palliative care makes care everyone's responsibility. Moreover, this approach identifies every single person as worthy of that care *irrespective of their lifestyle or circumstance*.[1] Although some forms of inequality and access are now widely debated and are public policy challenges to be reckoned with, the same cannot be said for the poor, homeless and substance-using publics. An informed national dialogue – one that leads to a more inclusive set of policies and an increasingly more compassionate set of practices for *these* people – is essential. These are the hopes behind every single chapter in this book.

Professor Allan Kellehear
University of Vermont, USA

Note

1   J. Abel & A. Kellehear [eds] (2022) *Oxford Textbook of Public Health Palliative Care*. Oxford University Press, Oxford.

Preface

This book has been written for people from health and social care who work on the front line of services, for those who manage or commission services, and those who develop and implement policy. Its focus is on people using substances, people who are in need of palliative or end-of-life care and people who have multiple needs requiring effective social and health care support. It moves away from purely biomedical perspectives and examines palliative and end-of-life care and substance use within a wider context of complex social and health care needs.

Its key aims are to:

1   Present what is known about the social and health care needs of different groups of people facing palliative or end-of-life care, who have a history of substance use. This includes the family members and friendship networks of people with lived experience.
2   Examine the intersectional marginalisation of different groups of people within a context of substance use at the end of life.
3   Discuss the very real challenges facing people at the end of life who use substances and how professional responses and health and social care system inequalities can impact upon them.
4   Present empirically based and practice-based evidence in a form that is informative, rigorous and useful for practice development.
5   Support the knowledge and practice of the readership through the use of case studies, offering ways to apply such knowledge to their work.

The origins of this book are rooted in a two-year research programme on end-of-life care for people using substances (alcohol and other drugs). Funded by the National Lottery Community Fund between 2016 and 2019, the research programme was the first of its kind to explore current practice and service experience from a range of perspectives. It was inspired by practitioners' concerns about improving the palliative and end-of-life care offered to people using substances, and their families, friends and carers. Professor Sarah Galvani and a team of researchers set about uncovering what was known about these issues. The team worked with three hospices and two substance use services across the North-West and Midlands regions of England, a regional community voices organisation, a project advisory group (comprising regional service commissioners; national charities and key people working in this field) and also an advisory group of people with lived experience (PWEs) who had histories of substance use or had been involved in palliative or end-of-life care. The research examined current knowledge and practice from a range of perspectives, including:

1 A review of published national and international research evidence.
2 Interviews with key informants in policy or practice roles whose work covered the overlap between substance use and end-of-life care.
3 A review of national datasets that might help determine the scale of the issue.
4 Interviews with people who used substances and were approaching the end of their life.
5 Interviews with families and carers of people who used substances and who were approaching the end of their life or had died.
6 Surveys and interviews with hospice and substance use service practitioners to gauge their experience of working with this client group, the challenges they faced and to document examples of good practice.

The motivation for this book stemmed from the degree of interest shown in the original research both nationally and internationally. This interest came primarily from practitioners, policy makers and other academics across the social and health care sectors. It attracted interest from practitioners in a range of specialist areas including substance use, mental health, palliative and end-of-life care, physical health to name a few.

What was notable about this interest were the synergies between people's experiences regardless of discipline or specialist area of practice, as well as their thirst for more information and knowledge. It was blatantly clear that people did not experience one disadvantage or belong to one marginalised group of people; rather they suffered multiple disadvantages in their lives and their attempts to access care. This intersectional marginalisation will be reflected in this edited collection.

A common factor in our research findings was the complexity of people's needs and the challenges this posed for practitioner responses in the absence of clear care pathways and joint working arrangements. Their call for more information and some guidance for practice are key drivers for this project. We were also aware that our original research missed out on some key factors at both individual and environmental levels, for example, greater inclusion of people from BAME (Black, Asian and Minority Ethnic) groups, or people in the criminal justice system. This book is an attempt to start filling these gaps.

Acknowledgements

We would like to thank the people who made the research underpinning these chapters possible. Particular thanks go to the individuals and family members who gave their time so willingly to participate in the research which provided the groundwork for some of these chapters. People spoke to us even when they had little time left to live or, as a family member or friend, were experiencing loss, grief and bereavement. Thank you for your honesty and courage.

We pay tribute to the practitioners who contributed to this book and those who contributed to research within it. At a time of stress and pressure in social and health care, resulting from austerity and then COVID-19, the practitioners offered their precious time and a willingness to take part.

We thank the authors of the chapters in this book for persevering through the Covid-19 pandemic and delivering their chapters to each deadline we set. We are lucky to have had such a talented group of contributors to work with.

Finally, we'd like to thank Grace at Routledge for her guidance and flexibility.

1   Introduction

Gary Witham, Sam Wright and Sarah Galvani

Definitions and terminology

Palliative care can be defined using a combination of the World Health Organisation (WHO) guidelines and part of a definition used by the European Association of Palliative Care (EAPC):

> Palliative care is an approach that improves the quality of life of patients and service users facing the problems associated with life-threatening illness, through the prevention and relief of suffering by means of early identification and assessment and treatment of pain and other problems, physical, psychological and existential. It also provides care to family members, friends and carers of patients and service users to recognise their need for support in their own right as well as to support them to care for their relative or loved one. Palliative care affirms life and regards dying as a normal process; it neither hastens nor postpones death. It sets out to preserve the best possible quality of life until death.

The definition of end of life varies according to role and perspective. For people working in palliative and end-of-life care, it can mean the last days or weeks of life. For others it relates to the last 12 months of life (General Medical Council (GMC, 2010). End of life can be difficult to predict within the context of chronic conditions, and substance use can make this even more challenging. Within the wider current literature there remains some ambiguity about the difference between the two, with authors using the terms interchangeably. Consequently, there is some inter-related use of the terms 'end of life' and 'palliative' in this book – although the term 'end of life' usually relates to the last 12 months of life (GMC, 2010).

Substance use is defined as current or previous alcohol or other drug use (prescribed or illicit). Within this book there are references to 'co-existing' conditions or 'dual diagnoses'. These terms are often used to describe a cohort of people who use drugs and/or alcohol and have other chronic conditions such as mental illness (for example, schizophrenia, severe depression or bi-polar disorder). Yet it is important to acknowledge that people are often not located statically in any category, but rather live with inter-related and constantly fluctuating co-existing

DOI: 10.4324/9781003187882-1

conditions. The impact of these on themselves and others caring for them is partly dependent on variables such as economic, social or health-related factors.

There is also an ongoing debate about terms used to describe people like 'patient' vs 'service user' or 'client' or 'person with lived experience'. Christmas and Sweeney (2016), for example, suggest 'patient' is a universal term for all people implying equality whereas 'service users' are automatically identified as using a formal service related to a specific illness/condition by virtue of their collective noun. Yet 'patient' automatically implies involvement with a health service and, in our thinking which is equally concerned with social care input, that is too limiting. So, within this book the authors have used a variety of these terms and this often reflects their professional background and the general lack of consensus in relation to current terminology.

Background

There has been a recent increase in people continuing to use substances into older age. As a result, people are living and dying with both substance use and related or unrelated chronic health conditions (Crome et al., 2018). Simultaneously, there has also been an increasing awareness of the inequitable access to end-of-life care globally (Stajduhar et al., 2020) with only an estimated 14% of the population who need palliative or end-of-life care receiving it (WHO, 2020). This combination of an ageing population using substances and living longer with chronic ill health poses significant challenges for the provision of palliative and end-of-life care. Barriers to effective end-of-life care include organisational factors that do not take account of structural inequalities within palliative care delivery, a lack of effective, evidence-based policies and educational programmes, and poor engagement with family members or peoples' social networks (Giesbrecht et al., 2018, Stajduhar et al., 2019, 2020). This situation requires care to move beyond a reliance on specialist provision and to be planned and delivered by a range of social and health care professionals.

The Rapid Evidence Assessment (REA) conducted by Witham et al. (2019b) examined end-of-life care for people with alcohol and other drug problems. Across the literature, which largely emanated from the USA, Canada and the UK, three major end-of-life themes were identified. These were: pain management, homelessness and marginalised populations, and alcohol-related death. In relation to pain management, there were persistent issues of under-treatment of pain for people using substances at the end of life. This often derived from fear among prescribing practitioners of overdosing their patient or professionals' assumptions about 'drug seeking' behaviours from people using substances. Prescribing outside standard pain management protocols also causes challenges for practitioners working in palliative care (Witham et al., 2019a, Merlin et al., 2020, Flaherty et al., 2021). This may be needed due to a high opioid tolerance among people with a previous history of opioid use. Support for comprehensive health assessment was evident within most papers in the REA to manage pain effectively and identify those people who needed this additional support. The literature appears to oscillate between focussing on abstinence and harm reduction, with surveillance of substance use at the end of life presented as a way of promoting safer opioid use. Yet, as several of the chapters of this book highlight, many people find it uncomfortable to talk about their substance use with health professionals – due to a fear of being judged and feeling stigmatised. Helping people to feel confident enough to disclose their substance use requires engagement skills and patience on behalf of the care professional.

Substance use at the end of life for people who are homeless or precariously housed is a topic with an increasing evidence base. Substance use is common among this population with Schneider & Dosani (2021) noting 61.9% of their homeless sample used substances. There has been an emphasis on examining the gaps in service provision for this population and the need to develop end-of-life care which may be shelter based rather than home or hospice (McNeil & Guirguis-Younger, 2012a). Many homeless services focus on recovery from addiction, which leaves talk about dying a secondary concern, thereby limiting opportunity for engagement (Shulman et al., 2018). The difficulty of recognising dying in this population also creates uncertainty over when to begin conversations related to advance care planning (care planning that takes account of end-of-life wishes). Research examining hospital-based experiences of end-of-life care among people who are homeless revealed their perceptions of hospital care as being inflexible and paternalistic, with their substance use hindering adequate care (Klop et al., 2018, Veer et al., 2018). This tended to lead to late presentation of severe symptoms in formalised care, with palliative care settings viewed as places to die and to be avoided. Given such significant structural barriers to accessing palliative or end-of-life care, it is crucial that services are flexible and proactively engage with shelters and other non-traditional settings to create joined up care and prevent a siloed system (Stajduhar et al., 2019).

Papers identified in the REA that related to alcohol focussed on cancer and liver cirrhosis. Problematic alcohol use appeared more common in younger palliative populations who had usually been referred late to end-of-life services (Kwon et al., 2013). Most papers focussed on the need for routine screening. For example, MacCormac (2017) asserts that screening is important since there is an increased tendency for people using alcohol to experience terminal agitation, high levels of comorbidities and poor social support at end of life. Mercadante et al. (2017) also refer to significant symptoms among people for whom screening indicates a potential alcohol problem and the need to refer early to palliative and end-of-life care services.

Implications for practitioners

As the chapters in this book reveal, the small but growing number of people using substances are now reaching an age when they may be dying from other chronic conditions. This poses numerous challenges for services and individual health and social care practitioners. Given some of the complexity of this population's needs, providing support often requires bespoke care. Yet when confronted with limited resources, effective, focussed interventions by health and social care prac-titioners can be difficult. This difficulty can further increase the marginalisation of this population as their complex needs require personalised care from multiple services, often at the last minute – which precludes much forward planning.

Since there is limited current evidence, we have no accurate way of assessing how significant the problem of substance use is in relation to advanced disease and end-of-life care. But it is reasonable to anticipate that it is a growing challenge which, when you add in the impact upon family caregivers and the stigma that they often feel, adds up to a significant group of affected people. It is, therefore, important for practitioners to identify and assess substance use by people referred to, or using, palliative or end-of-life care services. Families also need to be sup-ported through the needs assessment and care planning process. Substance use is particularly high among some clinical populations, for example, people with advanced head and neck cancers (Mercadante et al., 2017; Giusti et al., 2018). Therefore, proactively screening and identifying these problems is an important first step, followed by a knowledgeable, sensitive and informed practice response for the person and the family or friends providing care.

Local multi-disciplinary partnerships and effective joint working are important areas to develop to support people using substances at, or near, the end of life. This should be underpinned by better training and education for all health and social care practitioners on substance use and end-of-life care and extend to other support workers, such as staff in homeless shelters who are likely to engage with people using substances. Services also need to be flexible in providing end-of-life care in non-traditional contexts within a range of accommodation types.

Book structure

This book is structured in three parts. Part I explores different voices and ex-amines substance use at the end of life, with chapters from the perspectives of people using substances at the end of life, family members and health and social care practitioners. Part II examines health inequalities, with chapters exploring health literacy and the impact this has within the context of substance use at the end of life, the intersection of mental ill health and substance use, and finally a chapter exploring injecting drug use within the context of end-of-life care. Part III examines social inequalities with chapters relating to homelessness, vulnerable women and sex work, minority ethnic communities and finally a chapter examin-ing people in prisoner, substance use and the end of life.

Although issues of marginalisation, health and social inequalities often inter-sect, we have presented them in more discreet, separate categories. This is partly because we wish to clearly highlight the individual populations or marginalised communities, but also because this helps to make explicit those underlining commonalities between, for example, people using substances at the end of life who have mental health problems or learning disabilities, and people from black and minority ethnic groups or sex workers. This artificial separation into specific groups does not deny the diverse experiences of people using substances at the end of life. Yet it remains problematic for us as editors, not least when the main point we wish to make through this book is about the integration of service approaches. We hope that in highlighting support needs through a detailed, systematic approach, the common challenges between communities and populations can prompt health and social care provision to engage with what effective care looks like.

Intersectionality

While the origins of this book lie in the research on substance use and palliative and end-of-life care, there are many additional characteristics of individuals and groups that can further add to their marginalisation and the challenges for services to reach them. This book, therefore, adopts a lens of intersectionality and uses that to explore individual and systemic responses to people at end of life where there is, or has been, use of substances. Intersectionality has often been ill-defined (Hancock, 2007), however, germane to this paradigm are some central tenets that typify this approach (see Box 1.1).

As Hankivsky (2012) comments: 'according to an intersectionality perspective, inequities are never the result of single, distinct factors. Rather, they are the outcome of intersections of different social locations, power relations and experiences (p. 2)'. Within this book there are case studies that act as exemplars, highlighting the multiple ways in which inequalities can impact health and well-being for people using substances at the end of life. It is this complexity that can challenge appropriate practitioner support by often extending beyond an individual practitioner's expertise or that of the service provider.

On a more personal note, we encourage you, the reader, to engage wholeheartedly with this material – to absorb and feel these end-of-life experiences, many of

---

Box 1.1 Central tenets to intersectionality

- Human lives and experiences cannot be defined or reduced to single characteristics or factors.
- Social categories like race/ethnicity, class, ability and gender are socially constructed and open to challenge.
- How we construct our lives now and the context of our lives shapes our human experience.
- This process is mediated by our networks, wider social processes and structures.
- The influence of time and place is important and defined by power.
- The promotion of social justice and equity is a central tenet of intersectionality.

Hankivsky (2012); Hankivsky and Cormier (2009)

which may be very different from our own lives. With little or no direct contact with some of the people and contexts described in our chapters to draw upon, we tend to subconsciously distance ourselves from the distress these insights provoke in us. We may be prone to feelings of sympathy or pity, or our unconscious bias may tap into negative stereotypes and judgemental social learning that objectifies and stigmatises the people described in this book. So, it is crucial that we stay alert to these tendencies and consciously engage our reflective, compassionate selves. Through active 'listening' and paying careful attention to our emotions, we can examine and develop our compassionate responses.

References

Christmas, D., Sweeney, A. (2016) Service user, patient, survivor or client… has the time come to return to 'patient'? *British Journal of Psychiatry,* 209(1), 9–13. DOI: 10.1192/bjp.bp.115.167221

Crome, I., Dar, K., Jankiewicz, S., Rao, T., Tarbuck, A. (2018) *Our invisible addicts (College Report 2nd edition CR211).* London: Royal College of Psychiatrists. Retrieved: https://www.rcpsych.ac.uk/docs/default-source/improving-care/better-mh-policy/college-reports/college-report-cr211.pdf?sfvrsn=820fe4bc_2

de Veer, A. J. E., Stringer, B., van Meijel, B., Verkaik, R., Francke, A. L. (2018) Access to palliative care for homeless people: complex lives, complex care. *BMC Palliative Care,* 17, 119. DOI: 10.1186/s12904-018-0368-3.

Flaherty, A., Hossain, F., Vercelli, A. (2021) Meeting at the crossroads of pain and addiction: an ethical analysis of pain management with palliative care for individuals with substance use disorders. *Journal of Opioid Management,* 17(3), 207–214. DOI: 10.5055/jom.2021.0631. PMID: 34259332.

General Medical Council. (2010) *Treatment and care towards the end of life: good practice in decision making.* Retrieved March 2022 from https://www.gmc-uk.org/ethical-guidance/ethical-guidance-for-doctors/treatment-and-care-towards-the-end-of-life

Giesbrecht, M. A., Stajduhar, K. I., Mollison, A., Pauly, B., Reimer-Kirkham, S., McNeil, R., Wallace, B., Dosani, N., Rose, C. (2018) Hospitals, clinics and palliative care units: place-based experiences of formal healthcare settings by people experiencing structural vulnerability at the end-of-life. *Health & Place,* 53, 43–51. DOI: 10.1016/j.healthplace.2018.06.005

Giusti, R., Mazzotta, M., Venn, L., Sperduti, I., Di Pietro, F. R., Marchetti, P., Porzio, G. (2019) The incidence of Alcoholism in patients with advanced cancer receiving active treatment in two tertiary care centres in Italy. *Alcohol & Alcoholism,* 54(1), 47–50. DOI: 10.1093/alcalc/agy070

Hancock, A. M. (2007) Intersectionality as a normative and empirical paradigm. *Politics and Gender,* 3(2), 248–253. DOI: 10.1017/S1743923X07000062

Hankivsky, O. (Ed.) (2012) *An intersectionality-based policy analysis framework.* Vancouver, BC: Institute for Intersectionality Research and Policy, Simon Fraser University. https://data2.unhcr.org/en/documents/download/46176

Hankivsky, O. and Cormier, R. (2011) Intersectionality and public policy: some lessons from existing models. *Political Research Quarterly,* 64(1), 217–229. DOI: 10.1177/1065912910376385

Klop, H. T., de Veer, A. J., van Dongen, S. I., Francke, A. L., Rietjens, J. A. C., Onwuteaka-Philipsen, B. D. (2018) Palliative care for homeless people: a systematic review of the concerns, care needs and preferences and the barriers and facilitators for providing palliative care. *BMC Palliative Care*, 17(1), 67. DOI: 10.1186/s12904-018-0320-6

Kwon, J. H., Hui, D., Chisholm, G., Ha, C., Yennurajalingam, S., Kang, J. H., Bruera, E. (2013) Clinical characteristics of cancer patients referred early to supportive and palliative care. *Journal of Palliative Medicine*, 16(2), 148–155. DOI: 10.1089/jpm.2012.0344.

MacCormac, A. (2017) Alcohol dependence in Palliative Care: a review of the current Literature. *Journal of Palliative Care*, 32(3–4). DOI: 10.1177/0825859717738445

McNeil, R., and Guirguis-Younger, M. (2012) Harm reduction and palliative care: is there a role for supervised drug consumption services? *Journal of Palliative Care*, 28(3), 175–177. DOI: 10.1177/082585971202800308

Mercadante, S., Adile, C., Ferrera, P., Casuccio, A. (2017) The effects of alcoholism and smoking on advanced cancer patients admitted to an acute supportive/palliative care unit. *Supportive Care in Cancer*, 25(7), 2147–2153. DOI: 10.1007/s00520-017-3620-0

Merlin, J. S., Young, S. R., Arnold, R., Bulls, H. W., Childers, J., Gauthier, L., Giannitrapani, K. F., Kavalieratos, D., Schenker, Y., Wilson, J. D., Liebschutz, J. M. (2020) Managing opioids, including misuse and addiction, in patients with serious illness in ambulatory palliative care: a qualitative study. *American Journal of Hospice & Palliative Medicine*, 37(7), 507–513. DOI: 10.1177/1049909119890556.

Schneider, E., and Dosani, N. (2021) Retrospective study of a Toronto based Palliative care program for Individuals experiencing homelessness. *Journal of Palliative Medicine*, 1232–1235. DOI: 10.1089/jpm.2020.0772

Shulman, C., Hudson, B. F., Low, J., Hewett, N., Daley, J., Kennedy, P., Davis, S., Brophy, N., Howard, D., Vivat, B., Stone, P. (2018) A qualitative analysis explaining the challenges to access and provision of palliative care. *Palliative Medicine*, 32(1), 36–45. DOI: 10.1177/0269216317717101

Stajduhar, K. I., Giesbrecht, M., Mollison, A., Dosani, N., McNeil, R. (2020) Caregiving at the margins: an ethnographic exploration of family caregivers experiences providing care for structurally vulnerable populations at the end-of-life. *Palliative Medicine*, 34(7), 946–953. DOI: 10.1177/0269216320917875

Stajduhar, K. I., Mollison, A., Giesbrecht, M., McNeil, R., Pauly, B., Reimer-Kirkham, S., Dosani, N., Wallace, B., Showler, G., Meagher, C., Kvakic, K., Gleave, D., Teal, T., Rose, C., Showler, C., Rounds, K. (2019) *"Just too busy living in the moment and surviving"*: barriers to accessing health care for structurally vulnerable populations at end-of-life. *BMC Palliative Care*, 18, 11. DOI: 10.1186/s12904-019-0396-7

Witham, G., Peacock, M., Galvani, S. (2019a) End of life care for people with alcohol and drug problems: findings from a rapid evidence assessment. *Health and Social Care in the Community*, 27(5), e637–e650. DOI: 10.1111/hsc.12807

Witham, G., Yarwood, G., Wright, S., Galvani, S. (2019b) An ethical exploration of the narratives surrounding substance use and pain management at the end of life: a discussion paper. *Nursing Ethics*, 27(5), 1344–1354. DOI:10.1177/0969733019871685

World Health Organisation. (2020) *Palliative care.* https://www.who.int/news-room/factsheets/detail/palliative-care

Part I

Different voices

Introduction by Gary Witham

The chapters contained in Part I of this book focus primarily on the voices of those who use substances at, or near, the end of life, and the practitioners and family or friends who support them through this process. These chapters present empirical data generated from a research programme funded by the National Lottery Community Fund (see Preface). These chapters provide a foundation to further explore health and social inequalities developed in Parts II and III. In particular, Chapter 2 examines the experiences of people using substances at the end of life highlighting the stigma and stereotyping that often occurs when this population engage with formalised services. This can result in a reluctance to seek help and support by people using substances and subsequently, symptoms such as pain, tend to be poorly managed at the end of life. Chapter 3 focusses on the perspectives of health and social care practitioners and suggests that effective pain management can be challenging since practitioners are reluctant to use appropriate levels of opioid medications due to (unexplored) fears relating to opioid misuse. Training and partnership working for health and social practitioners are important elements in supporting people using substances particularly given their often-complex needs at the end of life and this is a significant thread throughout this section. The wider "siloed" care system further creates significant challenges in meeting the health and social care needs of this population due to the limited coordination of services. This can impact upon the place of care and the acknowledgement that different types of accommodation may be preferred by people using substances at the end of life such as hostels or shelters. Chapter 4 explores the dynamics between family and practitioner caregivers' and the sense of the uncertainty they share over the health prognosis of the person using substances. There was often a shared concern about doing something that was not helpful and the judgement associated with this but also a shared desire to provide for a "good" death that maintained dignity. The wider cultural context in which carers operated was also a challenge since they often felt stigmatised by their relative using substances and were cautious of the potential judgement by health and social care practitioners. This created problems with effective communication and was highlighted by all three of the chapters in this section. These chapters

DOI: 10.4324/9781003187882-2

offer an insight into different perspectives but often the same underlying problems are highlighted with stigma, discrimination and multiple complexity leading to poor experiences of people using substances, and their families at the end of life. Compassionate care, collaborative working and effective training are among some of the solutions articulated within these chapters. This should encourage reflective practice, professional curiosity and a desire to meet people where they are.

2 Death is not an abstract now

Approaching end of life as someone using substances

Sam Wright, Amanda Clayson and Jo Ashby

Introduction

Many people using alcohol and other drugs face substantial barriers in getting the right support to meet their end-of-life care needs, even when their substance use is in the past. As our larger end-of-life research project (Galvani, 2018) revealed, very little research, practice or policy work exists to inform the provision of palliative / end-of-life care for people who have current or historic substance use problems. They typically experience high degrees of both health and social inequalities, limiting their access to health and social care, which, in turn, reduces their chances of dying well. Using case studies, this chapter explores end-of-life care experiences among people using substances, their support needs and the implications that those needs pose for service provision.

After briefly describing the research that provided the basis for our ideas, this chapter is structured in three main sections, through which we:

1   Present the findings of our research and focus on two case studies of people approaching the end of their lives;
2   Discuss how their experiences of deprivation and stigma impair access to healthcare in general, and palliative/end-of-life care more specifically and
3   Consider the lessons that these people (and the wider participant cohort) provide for developing good, joined-up end-of-life practice and policy for people using substances and in need of palliative care.

Background literature

Problematic substance use has long been associated with premature death. To date, most UK policy focus has been on sudden, drug-related deaths (Corkery, 2008) and it is currently impossible to quantify the number of people who have both palliative care and substance use support needs (Webb et al., 2018). Yet this is a growing problem. Alcohol use is linked to 60 acute and chronic diseases and constitutes a leading risk factor for disease globally (Global Burden of Disease, 2016 Alcohol Collaborators, 2018), with 8,974 deaths related to alcohol-specific causes registered in the UK in 2020 (ONS, 2021). The number of people aged over

DOI: 10.4324/9781003187882-3

65 who use substances has grown in the UK over the past 20 years, and there is an ageing cohort of people using alcohol and drug treatment services (Royal College of Psychiatrists, 2018).

Structural inequalities and the social determinants of health

The lower a person's socio-economic situation, the worse their health is likely to be (Marmot, 2020). Substance use, associated as it is with both neighbourhood deprivation (PHE, 2016) and economic inactivity (ONS, 2017), exacerbates this. Alcohol-related mortality has risen significantly in England and Wales since the 1990s, disproportionately affecting people from disadvantaged socio-economic backgrounds, particularly women and men under 50 (Institute of Alcohol Studies, 2020). Men in the most deprived areas of England and Wales have a mortality rate 2.8 times higher than those in the least deprived areas; for women the rate is 2.1 times higher; for those who are homeless, use substances problematically, sell sex or have been in prison, the mortality rate is nearly eight times higher than the male average, and nearly 12 times higher for women (Aldridge et al., 2017).

The stigmatisation of people using substances

People with substance problems are stigmatised and marginalised in society (Rance et al., 2017). The raft of negative stereotypes about them (Radcliffe and Stevens, 2008) is further compounded by stigmatising attitudes towards the health, social care and housing problems that they commonly experience (Palepu et al., 2013). Social and healthcare practitioners may lack the education, training or support required to challenge these stereotypes or provide effective care for people who use substances (Van Boekel et al., 2013). This means that negative attitudes towards people who use substances are common because practitioners anticipate their healthcare delivery to be impeded by the person's poor motivation, manipulative behaviour and violence. Practitioners can also feel that people who have substance problems over-use resources, are not committed to improving their own health, do not take on health advice and are simply seeking drugs (Livingstone et al., 2012).

Suboptimal health and social care

Operating under such beliefs, health and social care practitioners may adopt more task-oriented approaches to their care, resulting in less personal engagement and diminished empathy with their patient, which, in turn, diminishes both the patients' feelings of empowerment and their subsequent treatment outcomes (van Boekel et al., 2013). This is an important aspect of people's poor engagement with healthcare services – perhaps rivalling the common depiction of people who use substances (particularly those considered to have 'chaotic lives') as not accessing healthcare due to simple logistical, physical or cognitive difficulties in keeping appointments. This was apparent in a study of 75 people who injected substances in Northern England. A range of practical and psychological barriers to accessing healthcare was discussed, but it was the stigmatising attitudes from professionals that particularly stood out (Neale et al., 2008).

How this relates to palliative and end-of-life care

There is a growing literature on palliative/end-of-life care for people who are homeless (Witham et al., 2019a) – many of whom use substances, have very poor physical and mental health and experience severe structural inequalities (Ebenau et al., 2019, 2020; Stajduhar et al., 2019; see Brophy and Colclough, 2022 in this book). Like other marginalised groups, there are two linked issues: (1) a lack of primary care, resulting in (2) late palliative care (if any) and consequent lost opportunity for Advance Care Planning (ACP) to improve quality of life. Until recently this has been framed in terms of individuals who are reluctant to engage with health services – but now there is growing recognition that health services are not designed to be inclusive of this population's needs.

What we know from the research conducted with people who are homeless and use substances is that even talking about palliative care is challenging. In their research in the Netherlands, Ebenau et al. (2019) have highlighted two key individual-level barriers for people who are homeless: (1) their closed or avoidant communication patterns, (2) and the extent to which their end-of-life preferences, coping-strategies and support needs differ from professionally accepted ideas and practices. From a structural perspective, Ebenau et al. (2020) described fragmented care, a lack of practitioner knowledge about the multiple challenges faced by people who are homeless, and insufficient time for practitioners to address them.

In Canada, Stajduhar et al. (2019), again researching people who are homeless and use substances, have identified five significant barriers to accessing care at end of life (EoL) which can easily be applied to people using substances:

1 The survival imperative;
2 The normalisation of dying;
3 The problem of identification;
4 Professional risk and safety management and
5 The cracks of a 'silo-ed' care system.

But what about people who are not homeless, whose substance use spans the spectrum from heavy social to harmful patterns of use? Palliative care in the UK has seen a great shift in prioritising more equitable access to good end-of-life care (EoLC) over the past ten years. Alongside this has been recognition of the importance of practitioners' compassion in engaging people from marginalised populations (St Mungo's and Marie Curie, 2011; Care Quality Commission and Faculty for Homeless and Inclusion Health, 2017). Yet, despite UK government policy proposing to provide high quality palliative care to all people who need it (Department of Health, 2008), consideration of the needs of people approaching the end of their life with alcohol/other drug problems remains absent from research and policy (Witham et al., 2018). Hence the need for our study, focussing as it does on the broader population of people who use substances – alcohol as well as other drugs.

The end-of-life care for people using substances study

This multi-disciplinary research project, funded by the National Lottery Community Fund, comprised six strands of work (Galvani, 2018). One strand involved in-depth, semi-structured interviews with people who were approaching the end of their life and were using or had used substances. Its aims were to:

1   Document how substance use and EoL services supported people with substance problems and terminal illness;
2   Report the good practice and challenges that people faced in accessing services and
3   Provide an opportunity for people reaching the end of their lives to comment on how support could be improved.

Albeit a challenging project, we had the privilege of being able to interview 11 people: seven men and four women, aged between 38 and 71 years old. They were accessed through the project's research partners: three hospices (four participants), two substance use services (three participants) and our community research partner, VoiceBox Inc., that identified people who were not using either palliative or substance use services (four participants).

Introducing our case studies

The two people we focus on for this chapter (Figure 2.1 and Figure 2.2) were selected purposefully to highlight some of the complex, materially and socially

---

Case study 1: Nigel, 55 years

Towards the end of his interview Nigel explained his perspective on why he felt he did not deserve attention around his own healthcare needs or even a say in what services are available:

> I'm one person out of a million drug addicts or alcoholics, you know. I'm just one cog in the wheel. I'm not that important: nothing special about me. There's millions worse off than me. I'm pretty lucky. I've got a roof over my head, I've got clean clothes, money in the bank. I'm not that important. … Maybe I'm just a bit lonely, sad - but there's so many people out there that really do need this [emotional support], they're the ones that are deserving more than me.

Nigel's case study above presents a familiar theme that occurred across all 11 research participants: that is, how access to help and support was perceived and experienced individually. The nuances of his life present a series of overlapping challenges that mean he needs holistic support that responds to his role as a carer at home, his substance use and his health concerns. What was particularly momentous in Nigel's description of his life was the way in which he minimised his existence as 'nothing special' and indeed considered himself to be 'lucky'. More worryingly, Nigel positions himself as unimportant and undeserving of healthcare and emotional support compared to others who he perceives as more deserving. Nigel appears to be drawing on stereotypical notions of 'drug addicts' and 'alcoholics' that subsequently lead him to consider himself in a fortunate position of having a 'roof' over his head, 'clean clothes' and 'money in the bank'. This positioning can be considered as positive from a mental health perspective. However, Nigel's position of feeling somehow unworthy of help, despite having significant health complications, could have negative consequences later if left unsupported.

Social care

- Nigel lives with his elderly mother and is her principle carer. Her health is declining and she has had a couple of recent hospital admissions where she could have died. She is increasingly dependent on Nigel, but they have no professional support. Nigel does not pay attention to his own health problems as he feels he needs to focus on caring for his mother who was a great support to him when his drug use was problematic.

Substance use

- Nigel is under the care of his local substance use team, receiving a buprenorphine prescription for opiate dependence. He has recently become involved with an informal men's group which provides peer emotional support and advice for older drug users who are typically experiencing lots of deaths among their social circles.

Health

- Nigel has several chronic physical health conditions including diabetes, COPD (diagnosed 10 years previously), cardiovascular disease and circulatory problems (associated with his diabetes). He is on medication for high blood pressure and valium for stress. He also has neuropathy in his left leg (linked to his diabetes) and can't walk far or exert himself without becoming out of breath.

Figure 2.1 The overlapping challenges facing Nigel.

deprived situations that many people using substances face at the end of their life. These brief case studies provide a helpful way of understanding substance use by giving insight into the daily realities of people's lives. Importantly, they encourage us to consider the multi-layered complexity of life; not just focussing on substance use or ill health but recognising shared experiences of the challenges of managing life and our common humanity.

Case study 2: Peter, 58 years

Peter's growing memory difficulties make him vulnerable to financial exploitation – experienced from both his daughter and his neighbour who used to 'knock round' when Peter was intoxicated to try to 'borrow' money for drugs. Peter's key worker had put a stop to both. But Peter's other concerns were his deteriorating health and his unmet social care needs – which he put down to being 'at the back of the queue' because of his previous alcohol problem:

Social care

- Until a year prior to interview, Peter had been living with his partner and her three small children. As his health started deteriorating, he left his partner and has since lived on his own. He has two adult daughters, one of whom was initially providing care for him. However, the carer allowance was removed from her over concerns that she was misusing her Dad's money and providing insufficient care. He now relies on a friend to help him whilst waiting for social care to be arranged.

Substance use

- Peter has been a heavy alcohol drinker throughout his adult life. He had periodically engaged with the local substance use service, and ceased drinking between 2011 and 2016. After a brief relapse a year prior to interview, he stopped drinking and started attending the substance use service again – although his poor mobility and memory problems prevent full engagement. His key worker undertakes home visits whenever he can.

Health

- Peter has had recurrent hospitalisations after being injured from falls due to peripheral neuropathy (nerve damage causing weakness and pain in hands and feet). He has recently been told that his liver is irreparably damaged, and has a second gastro-enterology appointment soon. His alcohol worker thinks Peter may either have had a stroke or be suffering from alcohol-related brain damage. His worker also thinks Peter should really be in a care home as his current care package is insufficient and fragmented.

Figure 2.2 The overlapping challenges of Peter's life.

A fortnight ago, the doctor discharged me from the hospital… And I just come home, I'm waiting for the hospital social worker and the physio … And still, up to today, I've still not spoke to the social worker or nothing… I haven't seen no-one. I've not got one answer of them. Still up to today. Seems as though they just push you out. Because I'm an alcoholic, they just put you at the back of the queue or whatever. But I'm not an alcoholic now, but I was a chronic alcoholic. I haven't touched it for 11 months … They're just treating me like a number. There's no more damage I can do, so they've just give up on me. It's two week ago that I asked for social services, but they've still not been in touch. It doesn't really matter how I feel does it? Because like I say, no one listens.

Anticipation of discrimination was a dominant theme described by all the participants in our research when they spoke about accessing healthcare or support. Dealing with stigmatisation and experiencing a lack of compassionate care was key in many experiences and is exemplified in Peter's account above. It was evident that although Peter had at the time of the interview, been sober for 11 months, he was nevertheless attributing his lack of care to his previous alcohol misuse. Despite his severe ill health he was not receiving any care to prepare him for a good death. Conversely, Peter talks about dehumanising experiences, being treated 'like a number', ignored and pushed out. Peter's account demonstrates the complexities and relational aspects of care that are brought about through power dynamics of healthcare professionals and the 'patient'. There is a real sense of Peter having no control over the last stages of life and not being heard in his plight for help. This fuels his sense of isolation – as experienced by many people with substance use problems – and moves Peter further away from experiencing a good death.

The two case studies (along with the reported experiences of the wider sample of research participants from whom they are drawn) reveal how problematic substance use presents an additional layer of disadvantage for people who are generally already experiencing multiple structural inequalities. Our research highlights that even when homelessness is not an issue, being outside the 'normative patient type' curtails people's access to healthcare, which often places palliative care services outside of their grasp.

One particularly strong aspect of this is the social and/or emotional isolation that can accompany substance use towards the end of a person's life. This is exemplified in Nigel's and Peter's case studies – compounded by feelings of not wanting attention or not 'deserving' care. The resulting late presentation to health services impedes access to palliative/EoL care, and in particular the chance to undertake advance care planning.

Moreover, in Peter and Nigel, we see two men who are not sure how ill they are. Their multiple health conditions, each of which in isolation may not be critical, in combination with their other conditions and their substance use leave them seriously (and unpredictably) ill. They have very limited informal support and little health or social care. For Nigel, this is because he prioritises caring for his frail mum, all the while believing that he does not deserve any attention. Peter, on the other hand, was desperate to know why he was experiencing periods of mental absence – but his memory and mobility problems make it almost impossible for him to get the support he needs. Indeed, although he was still in touch with his local substance use service, this was mainly thanks to his worker making unofficial outreach calls to overcome service inaccessibility. Yet, Peter's recovery worker had relatively little knowledge about his physical health and was also not sure how ill Peter was.

For Nigel and Peter we can discern a constellation of challenges – as presented in Figure 2.3 which highlights the intermingling complexity of people's lives and how that relates to their 'choices' around health:

Early symptoms of ill health are often 'masked' by substance use. Many people whose deaths are related to substance use have long histories of mental and physical ill health (Wright et al., 2017; Yarwood et al., 2018). Whether due to pre-existing health conditions, or simply becoming accustomed to the negative side effects of using alcohol and other drugs, people who use substances have often come to accept chronic ill health as 'normal'. In addition, substance use dulls perception of pain/illness, inhibiting recognition of how persistent or serious health

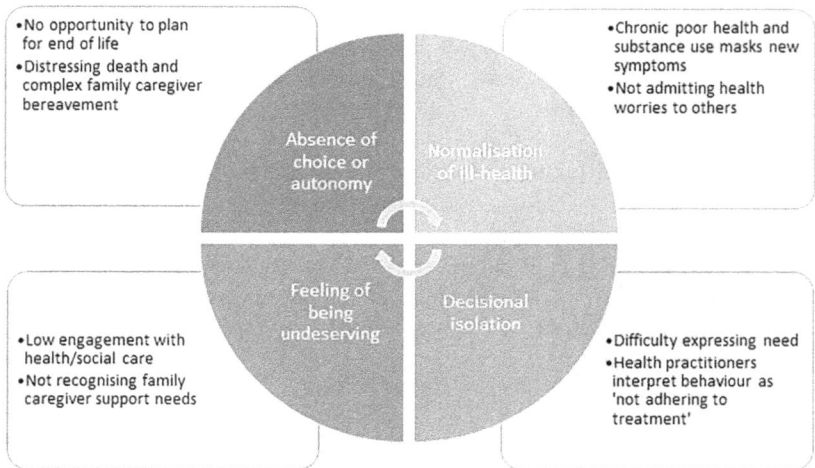

Figure 2.3 Key challenges facing people who use substances who have palliative care needs.

symptoms actually are. They may, therefore, be slow to consider the potential seriousness of new symptoms or seek a medical diagnosis.

Often through a combination of social isolation and wanting to avoid criticism about their substance use, many of the participants in our research did not discuss their health concerns with others. The shame, guilt and secrecy often associated with problematic substance use can result in a tendency to keep experiences, thoughts and feelings hidden. This was felt particularly in relation to seeking formal healthcare, where feelings of being unimportant or concerns over being judged as 'undeserving' resulted in low engagement with services and a tendency to defer decision-making to others.

Anticipation of health and social care practitioners' negative attitudes and potentially discriminatory behaviour can also result in late presentation to services (Ashby et al., 2018). Thus, we see how social isolation and absence of a trusting relationship with a health or social care practitioner can easily lead to low engagement with services, which may be interpreted as poor treatment adherence or a lack of motivation. The final parts of this trajectory involve the person lacking any choice or autonomy over care options while dying, resulting in them experiencing a potentially distressing death, and traumatic bereavement for the family, friends and carers left behind.

Thus, for people with substance use problems, approaching the end of life is arguably more challenging and less successful because of a variety of additional factors including:

- Health and social care practitioners may not communicate well or appropriately with them, for example, because of stigma;
- People with substance use problems may struggle to hear the message, due to anticipating discrimination, shutting down from judgemental authority figures or memory/capacity problems;
- People with substance use problems are likely to have limited family/carers around them to help absorb the information and
- They are more likely to be very close to death when presenting to healthcare services and need to make rapid care plans.

Our two case studies suggest an emotional layer that inhibits recognition of ill health and the accessing of care. This echoes Buchanan's assertion that: 'many problem drug users have had such limited options in life that they lack personal resources (confidence, social skills and life skills) and have limited positive life experiences to lean upon or return to' (Buchanan, 2004: 4). Worryingly, without any training about substance use, many healthcare practitioners know little about the psychological reasons that commonly lie behind it. Consequently, they interpret ongoing substance use as proof that the person does not care about their own health or 'deserve' treatment. Rather than simply framing problematic substance use as a 'choice' and a self-inflicted behaviour that warrants little sympathy, much greater understanding of people's life histories and their reasons for using substances would enable more trusting and compassionate relationships to form between people using substances and health/social care practitioners (Ashby et al., 2018).

In order to encourage more timely engagement with health and social care services, people using substances need to feel confident that they will not be judged harshly, through the filter of crude, negative stereotypes. They need to be assured that they will be met with compassion, understood as a 'whole person' with a challenging history, and that their healthcare needs will be responded to and prioritised – as for any other patient.

Indeed, if we consider problematic substance use as repeated behaviour to evade emotional distress or physical pain, then the need for greater prioritisation of emotional support for both the individual and their caregivers becomes clear, and the following cluster of actions need to be actioned:

1   Compassionate support and individually tailored engagement for each person;
2   Support for caregivers – either to existing caregivers (due to the long-term burden of care, their own substance use, and/or fractured relationships) or via the formation of a caring network, due to the absence of family and the likelihood of very personal and intimate care needs falling upon keyworkers and
3   Training and ongoing support to overturn negative stereotypes/stigmatisation among health and social care practitioners.

As Neale et al. (2008) have illustrated for people who inject drugs, Foucault's analyses of power provide a valuable lens through which to interpret why some health practitioners express negative attitudes over working with drug users. By seeing health practitioner and patient interactions as an exchange of power, whereby the professional dominates through wielding expert medical knowledge, diagnosing 'abnormality', and imposing treatment plans, we see clearly how practitioners 'have the power to marginalise or exclude clients whom they perceive as "difficult", "unsuitable" or "disruptive"' (Neale et al., 2008: 153).

People experiencing structural disadvantage can be highly attuned to these power dynamics, experiencing healthcare settings as oppressive, inflexible and demeaning (Giesbrecht et al., 2018). This greatly reduces their readiness to access services. So, if we are serious about eliminating barriers to healthcare and providing greater equity in access to palliative care, we need to focus on the quality of interactions between primary and acute healthcare staff – as gatekeepers to palliative care. We need to prioritise building practitioners' knowledge and understanding about (and compassion towards) people who use substances, to ensure that access to good palliative care (and healthcare more generally) is no longer contingent upon the client's perceived behaviour and that the professional's demeanour is put under a similar level of scrutiny.

The case studies we have presented reveal how people's experiences of intersectional marginalisation impact their end of life. We now turn to consider how health and social care responses can meet these challenges in terms of both practice and policy responses.

Practice and policy recommendations

Existing research literature provides key priorities for action. These include a need to: (1) improve recognition of substance use among palliative care patients and manage their pain more effectively (Mundt-Leach, 2016); (2) provide clinicians with training, support and planning resources to better identify older people using substances and their social, physical and other complex issues (RCPsych, 2018); and (3) adapt Advance Care Planning approaches to proactively address substance use and any potential complications, with integrated services to ensure effective care (RCPsych, 2018). Ebenau et al. (2020) recommend greater palliative care education among generic health and social care providers, supported by mobile specialist teams. They also highlight the need for support for caregivers and better integration between substance use, palliative and generalist healthcare. Our case studies and broader research provide additional evidence to support these recommendations.

Moreover, through our research we conclude that, for people using substances, the current medical referral pathway into palliative care that relies on identifying physical symptoms is too narrow an approach. Treatment is often delayed because of uncertainty over whether substance use is causing or exacerbating symptoms and because of the commonly held position that substance use needs to cease to clarify this. This can be broken down into three main problems:

1 Primary focus by medical professionals on physical symptoms alone, with reliance on a diagnosis which is obfuscated by substance use;
2 EoLC is initiated by medical diagnosis which excludes those outside of primary care and does not cater well for people with multiple chronic conditions and
3 EoLC requires patients' active engagement with medical institutions – excluding many people who have experienced trauma/stigma/discrimination.

Having identified some of the challenges arising from the multiple deprivation that people who use substances face and how professional responses can compound them, we propose six key recommendations for practice:

Practice recommendations

The priority is to bring about better identification of people who use substances and have severe, advancing ill health through systematic caseload review. This requires a broad range of health and social care practitioners feeling responsible for, and confident to act upon early concerns about the health and wellbeing of those they provide care to. This will enable:

1 Assertive and compassionate engagement, using psychologically informed approaches to understand the contextual and personal circumstances of each person. It will also facilitate earlier conversations about severe, advancing ill

health between people who use substances and trusted keyworkers. These keyworkers have a crucial role in supporting each person to navigate complex care systems and make decisions.

2   Parallel care planning that accepts uncertain health trajectories and that the person may continue to use substances. Care provision is not dependent on willingness to engage with explicit end-of-life conversations, but adapts to the readiness/capacity of the individual to plan ahead. Care needs to include (but not be dominated by) active treatment to avoid any substance use withdrawal **and** the offer of managed detoxification to anyone who wants it, as well as provision of timely treatment for new symptoms.

3   More diverse, flexible and appropriate health care settings that support better engagement and cater for multiple, complex healthcare needs. A broad range of health and social care organisations are needed to facilitate (and resource) the identification of people with serious advancing ill health that incorporates broader observations of behavioural change as a flag to provide specialist support. A multi-disciplinary case management approach that is sensitive to the cultural and power dynamics in interactions with health professionals could maximise the adaptability and availability of care (Giesbrecht et al., 2018).

Policy recommendations

The End-of-Life Care Strategy (Department of Health, 2008) and the NICE Quality Standard for End-of-Life Care (NICE, 2011, updated 2021) both aimed to enhance recognition of EoL conditions, increase referrals into EoLC services and improve care in the last year of life. In so doing, these policies sought to widen access to end-of-life care for people with non-cancer diagnoses and optimise choice over where people die. However, people with multiple morbidities and those living in deprived areas remain more likely to die in hospital than at home or in a specialist end-of-life care service, meaning that the gap in the equality of end-of-life care is actually widening (Higginson et al., 2017).

We need a national substance use policy shift to ensure that all health practitioners operate from a position of much greater understanding: accepting that ongoing substance use is likely (while offering access to treatment if that is desired) and providing healthcare and treatment plans which allow for that. To ensure that the infrastructure is in place to facilitate the development of good practice, we need to identify the challenges of, and potential solutions to, providing effective joined-up care (Galvani, 2018; Witham et al., 2019b). We therefore make the following three policy recommendations:

1   Make explicit a set of care values that promote social justice and commit to delivering equitable care for people who use substances. Discrimination against people who use substances needs to be eradicated, with all practitioners providing (and advocating for) compassionate health and social care.

2   Make better links across substance use and palliative/EoLC fields, so that palliative care approaches can be introduced as soon as the health of people

using substance use services causes concern to their key workers. Health care services need to gain consent to share pertinent information that facilitates flexible planning for people with complex health needs at the end of life.

3   Invest in ways to reach out to individuals at a community level to provide timely health care support, using a Community Recovery model or a Compassionate Community approach (Abel et al., 2018).

Recent theoretical analysis has shifted our understanding away from individual experiences of shame, to the political and economic 'weaponisation' of stigma as a means of excluding sections of the population from access to public resources (Tyler, 2020). Taking this perspective highlights how medical (individualist) healthcare models fail to address both health inequalities and their underlying social determinants, and so are in themselves a barrier to effective policy (Lynch, 2017). Thus, policies need to prioritise allocation of dedicated resources and better collaboration to facilitate both individual and structural interventions – for example: organisational measures to reduce deprivation; early intervention on adverse childhood experiences and service design that is guided by the views of people with experience to ensure inclusivity, equity and efficacy (Luchenski et al., 2018).

Conclusions

In this chapter, we have presented two case studies to highlight the complex situations and judgemental environment that people with substance problems typically face as they near the end of their lives. They highlight how intersectional marginalisation impedes people's access to end-of-life care, primarily through social isolation and self-stigma – resulting in people who use substances feeling that they do not deserve good healthcare. Thus, we see the cumulative impact of multiple deprivation at life's end. Moreover, we see that undignified and distressing death is not simply the product of the complex needs of people who are ill-suited to accessing, navigating and engaging with health and social care services. Rather, practitioners' attitudes and responses reflect and compound social inequalities within a system that commonly excludes the people most in need of care.

While substance use continues to be socially constructed as an individual 'flaw' – a 'lifestyle choice' – that renders people incapable or undeserving of care, little will change. Our practice and policy recommendations highlight the critical need for more relational and overtly compassionate approaches to support the meaningful provision of access to end-of-life care, in ways that genuinely engage with both people using substances and those caring for them. Accordingly, we – as a society – need to supplement our understanding of the 'social determinants of health' with the 'emotional determinants of access to care'. By doing so, we recognise substance use as *a consequence* of social exclusion, requiring greater empathy from health and social care practitioners – rather than being used as a means of justifying the withholding of compassionate care.

References

Abel, J., Kingston, H., Scally, A., Hartnoll, J., Hannam, G., Thomson-Moore, A., Kellehear, A. (2018) 'Reducing emergency hospital admissions: a population health complex intervention of an enhanced model of primary care and compassionate communities.' *British Journal of General Practice*, 68, (676), pp. e803–e810. DOI: 10.3399/bjgp18X699437

Aldridge, R., Story, A., Hwang, S., Nordentoft, M., Luchenski, S., Hartwell, G., Tweed, E., Lewer, D., Katikireddi, S., Hayward, A. (2017) 'Morbidity and mortality in homeless individuals, prisoners, sex workers, and individuals with substance use disorders in high-income countries: a systematic review and meta-analysis.' *Lancet*, 391, pp. 241–250. DOI: 10.1016/S0140-6736(17)31869-X

Ashby, J., Wright, S., Galvani, S. (2018) *End of life care for people with alcohol and other drug problems: interviews with people with end of life care needs who have substance problems.* Manchester, Manchester Metropolitan University. https://endoflifecaresubstanceuse.com/wp-content/uploads/2018/11/end-of-life-care-for-people-with-substance-use-family-report-phase-2-final-full-report1.pdf [Accessed 20th March 2022].

Brophy, N., Colclough, A. (2022) Homelessness and substance use within palliative and end-of-life care. In Witham, G., Galvani, S., Yarwood, G., Wright, S. (eds) *Substance use, end of life care and multiple deprivation: practice and research.* Oxon, Routledge.

Buchanan, J. (2004) 'Missing links? Problem drug use and social exclusion.' *Probation Journal*, 51 (4), pp. 387–397. DOI: 10.1177/0264550504048246

Care Quality Commission and Faculty for Homeless and Inclusion Health. (2017) *A second class ending: exploring the barriers and championing outstanding end of life care for people who are homeless.* https://www.cqc.org.uk/sites/default/files/20171031_a_second_class_ending.pdf [Accessed 4th March 2022].

Corkery, J. (2008) 'UK drug-related mortality - issues in definition and classification.' *Drugs & Alcohol Today*, 8 (2), pp. 17–25. DOI: 10.1108/17459265200800014

Department of Health. (2008) *End of life care strategy. Promoting high quality care for all adults at the end of life.* London, Department of Health. https://www.gov.uk/government/uploads/system/uploads/attachment_data/file/136431/End_of_life_strategy.pdf [Accessed 4th March 2022].

Ebenau, A., Dijkstra, B., ter Huume, C., Hasselaar, J., Vissers, K., Groot, M. (2019) 'Palliative care for people with substance use disorder and multiple problems: a qualitative study on experiences of patients and proxies.' *BMC Palliative Care*, 18, p. 56. DOI: 10.1186/s12904-019-0443-4

Ebenau, A., Dijkstra, B., ter Huurne, C., Hasselaar, J., Vissers, K., Groot, M. (2020) 'Palliative care for patients with substance use disorder and multiple problems: a qualitative study on experiences of healthcare professionals, volunteers and experts-by-experience.' *BMC Palliative Care*, 19, p. 8. DOI: 10.1186/s12904-019-0502-x

Galvani, S. (2018) *End of life care for people with alcohol and other drug problems: what we know and what we need to know. Final Project Report.* Manchester, Manchester Metropolitan University. http://e-space.mmu.ac.uk/622052/1/EOLC%20Final%20overview%20report%2027%20November%202018%20PRINT%20VERSION.pdf [Accessed 4th April 2019].

Giesbrecht, M., Stajduhar, K.I., Mollison, A., Pauly, B., Reimer-Kirkham, S., McNeil, R., Wallace, B., Dosani, N., Rose, C. (2018) 'Hospitals, clinics, and palliative care units: place-based experiences of formal healthcare settings by people experiencing structural vulnerability at the end-of-life.' *Health Place*, 53, pp. 43–51. Epub 2018 Jul 25. PMID: 30055467. DOI: 10.1016/j.healthplace.2018.06.005

Global Burden of Disease (GBD) 2016 Alcohol Collaborators. (2018) 'Alcohol use and burden for 195 countries and territories, 1990–2016: a systematic analysis for the Global Burden of Disease Study.' 2016. *Lancet*, 392, pp. 1015–1035. https://www.thelancet.com/action/showPdf?pii=S0140-6736%2818%2931310-2 [Accessed 23rd March 2022].

Higginson, I., Reilly, C., Bajwah, S., Costantini, M., Gao, W., on behalf of the GUIDE_Care project (2017) 'Which patients with advanced respiratory disease die in hospital? A 14 year population based study of trends and associated factors.' *BMC Medicine*, 15, p. 19. DOI: 10.1186/s12916-016-0776-2.

Institute of Alcohol Studies. (2020) *Alcohol and health inequalities.* https://www.ias.org.uk/wp-content/uploads/2020/12/Alcohol-and-health-inequalities.pdf [Accessed 30th November 2021].

Livingstone, J.D., Milne, T., Fang, M.L., Amari, E. (2012) 'The effectiveness of interventions for reducing stigma related to substance use disorders: a systematic review.' *Addiction*, 107, pp. 39–50. DOI: 10.1111/j.1360-0443.2011.03601.x

Luchenski, S., Maguire, N., Aldridge, R.W., Hayward, A., Story, A., Perri, P., Withers, J., Clint, S., Fitzpatrick, S., Hewett, N. (2018) 'What works in inclusion health: overview of effective interventions for marginalised and excluded populations.' *Lancet*, 391, pp. 266–280. DOI: 10.1016/S0140–6736(17)31959-1

Lynch, J. (2017) 'Reframing inequality? The health inequalities turn as a dangerous frame shift.' *Journal of Public Health*, 39 (4), pp. 653–660. DOI: 10.1093/pubmed/fdw140

Marmot, M., Allen, J., Boyce, T., Goldblatt, P., Morrison, J. (2020) *Health equity in England: The marmot review 10 years on.* London, Institute of Health Equity. https://www.health.org.uk/publications/reports/the-marmot-review-10-years-on [Accessed 4th March 2022].

Mundt-Leach, R. (2016) 'End of life and palliative care of patients with drug and alcohol addiction.' *Mental Health Practice* 20 (3), pp. 17–21. DOI: 10.7748/mhp.2016.e1148

National Institute for Health and Clinical Excellence. (NICE) (2011, updated 2021) *Quality standard for end of life care.* https://www.nice.org.uk/guidance/qs13/chapter/Quality-statements [Accessed 4th March 2022].

Neale, J., Tompkins, C., Sheard, L. (2008) 'Barriers to accessing generic health and social care services: a qualitative study of injecting drug users.' *Health and Social Care in the Community*, 16 (2), pp. 147–154. DOI: 10.1111/j.1365-2524.2007.00739.x

Office for National Statistics. (2017) *Statistics on drugs misuse: England, 2017.* London, ONS. http://www.content.digital.nhs.uk/catalogue/PUB23442 [Accessed 30th July 2018].

Office for National Statistics (ONS). (2021) *Alcohol-specific deaths in the UK: registered in 2020.* London, ONS. https://www.ons.gov.uk/peoplepopulationandcommunity/healthandsocialcare/causesofdeath/bulletins/alcoholrelateddeathsintheunitedkingdom/registeredin2020#alcohol-specific-deaths-in-the-uk [Accessed 23rd March 2022].

Palepu, A., Gadermann, A., Hubley, A., Farrell, S., Gogosis, E., Aubry, T., Hwang, S. (2013) 'Substance use and access to health care and addiction treatment among homeless and vulnerably housed persons in three Canadian cities.' *PLoS One*, 8 (10), p. e75133. Published online 2013 Oct 4. https://www.ncbi.nlm.nih.gov/pmc/articles/PMC3790780/ [Accessed 30th July 2018]. DOI: 10.1371/journal.pone.0075133

Public Health England. (2016) *The public health burden of alcohol and the effectiveness and cost-effectiveness of alcohol control policies: An evidence review.* London, PHE. https://www.gov.uk/government/publications/the-public-health-burden-of-alcohol-evidence-review [Accessed 4th March 2022].

Radcliffe, P., Stevens, A. (2008) 'Are drug treatment services only for 'thieving junkie scumbags'? Drug users and the management of stigmatised identities.' *Social Science & Medicine*, 67, pp. 1065–1073. DOI: 10.1016/j.socscimed.2008.06.004

Rance, J., Treloar, C., Fraser, S., Bryant, J., Rhodes, T. (2017) '"Don't think I'm going to leave you over it": accounts of changing hepatitis C status among couples who inject drugs.' *Drug and Alcohol Dependence*, 173, pp. 78–84. DOI: 10.1016/j.drugalcdep.2016.12.020

Royal College of Psychiatrists. (RCPsych) (2018) *Our invisible addicts*. 2nd edition College Report CR211. London, Royal College of Psychiatrists. https://www.rcpsych.ac.uk/docs/-default-source/improving-care/better-mh-policy/college-reports/college-report-cr211.pdf?sfvrsn=820fe4bc_2 [Accessed 27th September 2021].

St Mungo's and Marie Curie. (2011) *Supporting homeless people with advanced liver disease approaching the end of life*. https://www.mariecurie.org.uk/globalassets/media/documents/-commissioning-our-services/current-partnerships/st-mungos-supporting-homeless-may-11.pdf [Accessed 30th July 2018].

Stajduhar, K.I., Mollison, A., Giesbrecht, M., McNeil, R., Pauly, B., Reimer-Kirkham, S., Dosani, N., Wallace, B., Showler, G., Meagher, C., Kvakic, K., Gleave, D., Teal, T., Rose, C., Showler, C., Rounds, K. (2019) '"Just too busy living in the moment and surviving": barriers to accessing health care for structurally vulnerable populations at end-of-life.' *BMC Palliative Care*, 18, p. 11. DOI: 10.1186/s12904-019-0396-7

Tyler, I. (2020) *Stigma: the machinery of inequality*. London, Zed Books.

van Boekel, L.C., Brouwers, E., van Weeghel, J., Garretsen, H. (2013) 'Stigma among health professionals towards patients with substance use disorders and its consequences for healthcare delivery: systematic review.' *Drug and Alcohol Dependence*, 131, 1–2, pp. 23–35. DOI: 10.1016/j.drugalcdep.2013.02.018

Webb, L., Wright, S., Galvani, S. (2018) *End of life care for people with alcohol and other drug problems*. Report on Strand 2: scoping review of existing database evidence. Manchester, Manchester Metropolitan University. https://endoflifecaresubstanceuse.com/wp-content/uploads/2018/11/end-of-life-care-for-people-with-substance-use-existing-datasets-full-report.pdf [Accessed 20th March 2022].

Witham, G., Galvani, S., Peacock, M. (2018) *End of life care for people with alcohol and other drug problems: rapid evidence assessment*. Manchester, Manchester Metropolitan University. https://endoflifecaresubstanceuse.com/wp-content/uploads/2018/11/end-of-life-care-for-people-with-substance-use-rea-full-report-31-july-2018.pdf [Accessed 20th March 2022].

Witham, G., Peacock, M., Galvani, S. (2019a) 'End of life care for people with alcohol and drug problems: findings from a rapid evidence assessment.' *Health and Social Care in the Community*, 27 (5), pp. e637–e650. DOI: 10.1111/hsc.12807

Witham, G., Yarwood, G., Wright, S., Galvani, S. (2019b) An ethical exploration of the narratives surrounding substance use and pain management at the end of life: a discussion paper. *Nursing Ethics*. DOI: 10.1177/0261018320960009e

Wright, S., Yarwood, G., Templeton, L., Galvani, S. (2017) *End of life care for people with alcohol and other drug problems. Secondary analysis of interviews with family members, friends and carers bereaved through a relative's substance use*. Manchester, Manchester Metropolitan University. https://endoflifecaresubstanceuse.com/wp-content/uploads/2018/11/end-of-life-care-for-people-with-substance-use-family-strand-phase-1-report.pdf [Accessed 20th March 2022].

Yarwood, G., Wright, S., Templeton, L., Galvani, S. (2018) *End of life care for people with alcohol and other drug problems. Qualitative analysis of primary interviews with family members, friends and carers*. Manchester, Manchester Metropolitan University. https://endoflifecaresubstanceuse.com/wp-content/uploads/2018/11/end-of-life-care-for-people-with-substance-use-family-report-phase-2-final-full-report1.pdf [Accessed 20th March 2022].

3   Views from the coalface

Social and health care professionals working with people using substances at, or near, the end of their lives

Sarah Galvani, Cherilyn Dance and Sam Wright

Introduction

The social and health care professionals who work with people using substances at, or near, the end of their lives, straddle a multitude of disciplines. In this chapter, we draw on this breadth of knowledge across this range of professions. We present examples from their experiences of working with this group of people; people who are often marginalised and stigmatised due to their substance use, and who become defensive and cautious of service provision as a result.

People supported by this range of professionals may be using substances (alcohol or other drugs) until the last days of their lives. For others, their substance use may have been in the past, but could still be seen to impede their access to care and their relationships with family, friends and professionals. For some people, their substance use was directly related to the health condition from which they were dying – for example, alcohol-related liver disease. For others (often people using illicit drugs), there was no clear direct causation, but their use of illicit drugs exacerbated or complicated the social and health care response. Either way, substance use – whether current or in the past – often resulted in both self-stigmatisation and concern over being judged negatively by practitioners (Ashby et al., 2018). This can impair the ability of people using substances to get the palliative care they needed to achieve a peaceful and dignified death.

The data presented in this chapter are drawn from a research project exploring end-of-life care for people using substances based in England between 2016 and 2018. One strand of the research focussed on the experience of professionals working in substance use services and hospices, as well as a group of key informants (KIs) from a wide range of community or health care settings including liver specialists, social workers, GPs and coroners, among others. The KIs were not a random sample; but rather were selected as individuals or as representatives of agencies with particular knowledge of the palliative care needs of people who use substances. One substance use agency had run a specialist service for people with liver conditions and therefore had greater knowledge about, and engagement with, palliative services. One of the hospices was more familiar with caring for people with substance use histories due to its geographical location in the UK and the higher levels of substance use within the local population. Thus, the sample

DOI: 10.4324/9781003187882-4

for this research included professionals with more knowledge of these overlapping issues than might be expected among their peers.

Professionals from social and health care services need to be adequately prepared – not only for the sake of the people who access their services and their significant others, but equally for the sake of their own mental and emotional well-being. They need to be able to offer palliative care that responds to the social, emotional, spiritual and physical needs of people using substances. This chapter sets out two of the common practice challenges faced by these professionals: (i) pain and symptom management for people using substances and (ii) caring for people who do not want to stop using substances. It discusses the challenges, potential solutions and strategies to overcome them.

Research design

The findings presented here draw on the qualitative data collected using focus groups and individual interviews during the course of the research. Seventeen key informants were interviewed from around the UK: comprising community- and health-based practitioners as well as policymakers. To protect anonymity, the key informant participants have been grouped into similar professions and are cited in this chapter by their group membership, for example, Group 1 – Frontline SHCP (Social and Health Care Practitioners). In addition, 53 people participated in focus groups or individual interviews and are cited as such in this chapter: 25 were substance use practitioners and 28 were hospice practitioners. All the agencies were located in the North West of England except one which was based in the Midlands region. Data were analysed using a template approach to thematic analysis (Brooks and King, 2014). Template analysis incorporates two forms of analysis; the first, constructing an initial thematic template from an early reading of a selection of the data, acknowledges the focussed nature of questions and the selective data gleaned as a result; the second involves a more grounded, 'bottom up' approach of data analysis to allow additional themes to be identified. Combining both methods of analysis facilitates a transparency to the data collection and analysis process.

Pain and symptom management

Twenty-five of the papers in Witham et al.'s (2019) substance use and end-of-life care evidence review related specifically to pain and symptom management. Of those, 23 were authored in the USA, one in Canada and one in the UK. While there was a mix of evidence reviews, case studies and a small number of empirical studies, the majority highlighted the challenges of pain management for people using substances, particularly opiates (Chou et al., 2009; Passik et al., 2009; Taveros and Chuang, 2016). They also raised concerns about drug diversion as a result of prescribing practice (Krashin et al., 2012; Pancari and Baird, 2014). Further issues that need addressing included: under-prescribing practice leading to 'chemical coping,' that is, using substances on top of medication (Kwon et al., 2015), the need for ongoing screening (Kutzen, 2004; Tan et al., 2015), as well as the need for staff to have support and better training (Doukas, 2014).

A clear message from the health professionals involved in the research was the complication that ongoing substance use caused in terms of pain and symptom management (Galvani et al., 2018a). Given a core aim of palliative and end-of-life care is to maximise comfort and minimise pain (Witham et al., 2019), this presented a key challenge. As one hospice professional told us, "It certainly does affect how you manage their symptoms."

Professionals expressed fears about both over- and under-prescribing for pain:

> I think, generally speaking, there's a huge ignorance in managing pain in patients who are either current drug users or past drug users at end of life with cancer. There is a fear isn't there about prescribing?
>
> [Hospice professional – focus group]

The fear of over-prescribing was located in concerns about someone dying as a result of overdose. This fear, be it experienced by the prescriber or the administrator of the medication, threatened their professionalism and, ultimately, their job:

> Because you know, if you're the one that's administered it, you're responsible.
>
> [Hospice professional – focus group]

Some of this fear stemmed from not knowing exactly what the person had taken and how many people they had prescribing for them:

> We let the GP know. But if that patient's known to an oncologist or a heart specialist or a renal specialist and they also have community matron and they have a GP, you've potentially got four or five people who can prescribe.
>
> [Hospice professional – focus group]

These fears were reported, not only by hospice professionals, but also by community health practitioners, including pharmacists. Pharmacists' responses varied with some good partnership practice noted in relation to safe prescribing:

> We have some pharmacies that are very good, some pharmacies that are: 'No, we won't deliver to the hostel, sorry, they have to come down and pick it up'…when you do have great relationship with pharmacies who are really flexible and understanding and work well together, that usually comes down to having a compassionate or lovely pharmacist who managed a service, or somebody who is championing the cause of homeless people or people with substance use issues, rather than it being a blanket service level understanding of the need for flexibility with this client group.
>
> (Group 1- Frontline SHCP)

On the other hand, the fear of under prescribing and therefore leaving people in pain and needing to 'top up' their prescribed medication with illicit drugs was also a concern. This is referred to as "chemical coping" in the research literature (Kwon et al., 2015). One example of under-prescribing, provided by a hospice professional, was a woman with a history of substance use 12 years previously. She required increasing measures of morphine to counter her pain, but the GP was reluctant to prescribe it, requiring the professional to advocate with the GP on her behalf to ensure she had adequate pain control.

One of the challenges for health professionals was determining the tolerance levels of the individual to the prescribed medication. Someone with long-term use of illicit opioid drugs, for example, would have a far higher physical tolerance of opioid-based medication and it would therefore not be adequate to prescribe medication at the (lower) levels suggested by clinical guidelines. One of the hospice participants in the research described having to give very high doses of medication to someone with high tolerance levels before they noticed a reduction in their pain:

> I guess where we hear about things that are of concern clinically will be things like people being afraid to prescribe analgesia properly, particularly if somebody has a heroin or some kind of a drug related abuse... My clinical experience is that some people, particularly with heroin abuse or related drugs, have a very high tolerance for the drug and therefore they need really big doses... People are really afraid of really big doses and so I think that there is a tendency to underserve this population.
>
> (Group 3- Policy & Commissioning Professionals)

Professionals faced similar challenges with other prescribed drugs:

> ... I know that I struggled with thinking about the drugs and what to suggest prescribing. I mean if somebody's on so much Diazepam that they're taking, you know, what do you then do in terms of symptom management? How do you manage their anxiety when they're already taking shed loads of Diazepam?
>
> [Hospice professional – interviewee]

In addition to concerns about under and over prescribing, medicating people's pain and symptoms was also difficult when family or friends brought in alternative medications from the community:

> Myself and another colleague brought [a person] in ... his son had gone and got some under the counter medication for him. ... It was cannabis oil and what he'd done is actually because he thought that this also would make his dad better, because the chemo hadn't worked. In his mind, he'd been told that this was a cure... His dad, he stopped all his medication and we kept upping his medication. ...He died in here, but [the son] still couldn't get his head

round this, because he'd been told that this was a cure and he was absolutely fixated on it, thinking he was saving his daddy. But he'd not been taking his morphine probably for two weeks. He was in agony …

[Hospice professional – focus group]

Alcohol was a commonly cited 'painkiller' or anxiolytic that people took, although other more unusual substances were also reported (Galvani et al., 2018a). Professionals reported a range of herbs and spices being used, including cumin and turmeric. The key concerns, as identified in the quote above, were either the person stopping taking their prescribed medication and suffering as a result, or the unknown interaction of the new substance with the prescribed medication.

While this research focussed on people using substances, we also included people with historic substance use as we found similar concerns relating to their care at, or near, the end of their lives. Professionals told us of examples where people with past substance use were "so reluctant to consider painkillers again because they're so fearful" [Hospice professional – focus group].

Despite being at or near the end of their lives, people who have used substances in the past and fought hard to stop or reduce their substance use are often fearful of becoming dependent on them once more and/or experiencing withdrawal again:

I do have another lady on my caseload just now, who is an ex user. … She won't take the liquid morphine, she's terrified of taking it. She'll try and put up with the pain, because of that fear of addiction. …There is a fear if they've been clean for a while, there really is a fear of getting back on and that. It's like they feel they're going to lose total control of their lives.

[Hospice professional – focus group]

The key informant interviews highlighted how some people were concerned that their use of substances, and the level of it, would mean they would not get pain management at high enough levels:

… I just reassure them that the team will take [their drug use] into account and 'There won't be a limit on your pain relief.' And I think that stops people stockpiling as well – if you give guarantees that your pain relief will be the main focus, if you need higher amounts of drugs, you'll get them.

(Group 1- Frontline SHCP)

Some key informants raised concerns about double standards applied to people known to use substances and their reported levels of pain:

We talk about the pain…what the patient tells you it is. But that doesn't seem to apply to this group in terms of other people. So they're 'looking for drugs, they've asked for it four hourly.' Whereas, if it was a wee old lady who was 80 who was asking for extra painkiller, they'd be paging us going, 'She's really sore, you need to come and do something about it.'

(Group 2- Senior SHCP)

In spite of the challenges and fears faced by the professionals in relation to prescribing practice, some solutions were offered:

- One hospice invited the district nurses to the hospice to talk about prescriptions for people using substances "because if we just sent [the prescription] out, they would have fallen over when they saw that [quantity]" [Hospice professional – focus group].
- The palliative care consultant from one hospice visited a hospital to explain the person needed a higher dose because of their tolerance levels.
- Some hospice professionals found that directly questioning people about their substance use led to an open and direct response from the person. They were then able to change their medication management accordingly. These professionals pointed out that such information and advocacy facilitated better care when people returned to their homes in the community.

Other ideas included:

- Arranging with a chemist for the daily delivery of drugs to a person's home.
- Safe storage boxes for medications in the home.
- Arranging for a pub landlady to look after an isolated customer's 'just in case' medication "…because they were aware when he didn't come in [to the pub], so there are in-built support mechanisms from that" (Group 1- Front-line SHCP).

The need for education and training around supporting people using substances, prescribing doses, and different approaches that could be used to alleviate pain and anxiety was a theme raised repeatedly in the research. So too, was the need to have a good understanding of the patient and their multiple needs, alongside skilled and compassionate practice. One senior SHCP suggested that liver specialists could provide guidance for hospices around liver disease in particular. Existing guidance was not considered to be adequate as it did not directly address the overlapping issues of substance use and end-of-life care.

Caring for people who do not want to stop using substances

The literature relating to the second focus of this chapter: caring for people at the end of their lives who use substances, is minimal. Of the 60 papers in Witham et al.'s 2019 review, many adopted a clinical 'management' perspective based on reviews or case studies rather than presenting a more holistic care response. The evidence most closely linked with how to support, or work with, people using substances at, or near, the end of their lives, fell into a group of papers about homeless and marginalised people and palliative care. Fifteen of the 60 papers made reference to the need for improved access to end-of-life care, person-centred approaches and outreach to care in the community. They also highlighted the multiple disadvantages faced by this group of people and the need to consider such disadvantages in delivering palliative and end-of-life care. In sum, there was a call for a more compassionate and co-ordinated care response including greater flexibility around treatment compliance (Morgan et al., 2008; MacWilliams et al., 2014) and a harm reduction framing of their end-of-life care (McNeil and Guirguis-Younger, 2012).

Professionals spoke of the challenge of caring for people approaching the end of their lives who wanted to continue using substances (including alcohol). They discussed the extent to which they should be advocating for the person to change their substance use towards the end of their lives, rather than accept that at that stage of the person's life, there was little point in expecting them to change entrenched patterns of substance use. Some hospice practitioners clearly felt that pressuring people to change was not appropriate:

> I don't think being judgemental and trying to adjust or stop behaviour, that's been going on for decades in some cases, for somebody who's imminently dying, is appropriate.
>
> [Hospice professional – focus group]

Other professionals felt offering people the choice of change, even in the latter stages of their life was appropriate. However, it needed to be done by building relationships quickly in order to gain trust and have open conversations with people about their current and past substance use:

> I think it's building up a really good relationship so that they're honest with you and give them permission to be honest in terms of what they've taken, what they're taking now and explain that we're not going to be judgemental over that, we just want to establish it so that we can help them.
>
> [Hospice professional – interviewee]

One of the study's key informants spoke about the need to acknowledge when people did not want to change their substance use and continue to provide good care anyway. In his example, he had attempted to address a person's drinking and related liver disease with little success – as the person continued to drink heavily. At this point the professional changed his approach:

> … you don't ask them to stop drinking, you sort of take alcohol away [from the conversation] and say '…so now because this addiction is part of your illness, we need to start thinking about how we're going to plan the end of your life.'….You take away the, 'If you don't stop drinking, you'll die.'… and change the focus to: 'Drinking is part of your pathology. We need to deal with that in the same way as we need to deal with your liver chemistry.'
>
> (Group 2- Senior SHCP)

What this allows is a conversation about the person's wishes for the end of their life. However, for some substance use professionals, the challenge was talking to people about their wishes or plans for the end of their lives in the first place. Several practitioners spoke about the lack of training in asking about these issues, while another who had worked on an older people's project had more knowledge and experience and was more comfortable with asking about end-of-life care needs:

> I think our care planning does cover a lot of the health and wellbeing aspects of somebody's care. But at what stage that turns into an end-of-life conversation is a different thing and I don't think our staff are particularly... we haven't trained people in that area of work ….
>
> [Substance use professional – interviewee]

Similarly, some palliative and end-of-life care staff felt uncomfortable asking about substance use and the need for further awareness and skills was noted:

> It's about skilling them all up to be comfortable in, perhaps, asking those questions that perhaps are a bit more difficult to ask. So, for me, I think it's about … increasing awareness across the hospice.
>
> [Hospice professional – interviewee]

Where substance use is ongoing, people's health can deteriorate rapidly prior to death, so early conversation about their wishes for end-of-life care is important. Further, it can minimise the shock for both themselves and their family members, which is crucial to attend to – particularly if they had not been aware of their prognosis from previous contact with health staff (Ashby et al., 2018; Yarwood et al., 2018).

For substance use professionals, a person's ongoing substance use at, or near, the end of their lives was not unusual. Substance use professionals were accustomed to working with people who had multiple and complex needs alongside, or as a result of, their substance use and whose longevity was unpredictable. However, it is likely that these professionals saw only the 'tip of the iceberg' given people drop out of services when they become unwell, while most others do not engage with treatment in the first place.

Even when they advocated for their 'client,' their experience was often not recognised by other professionals:

> … we had a client who we could see was dying and he was going in and out of hospital, he was bouncing in and out with ascites* problems. And we asked [the GP] "Can't this person be returned to palliative care?" … and the GP said, "I can't refer to palliative care unless the consultant did." So I said: "Let's ask the consultant again." So I emailed the consultant. The consultant then told me, "This person is not palliative. This person needs to stop drinking." And he died three weeks later.
>
> [Substance use professional – focus group]

(*abnormal build-up of fluid in the abdomen)

The lack of empathy from some SHCPs towards people who continue to use substances in spite of a terminal health condition was familiar to substance professionals. Some practitioners who do not have much knowledge about substance use can be judgemental and assume that people do not 'deserve' treatment until they have stopped using alcohol or other drugs. The substance professionals interviewed for this research emphasised the need for empathy and understanding about what was potentially driving someone's continued use of substances even in the face of their imminent death:

> …it seems completely alien to us why somebody would drink themselves to death. But, when you understand the context of somebody's life and the things they've been through, it makes sense. And I suppose that's the really, very, very sad thing, you really do understand the struggles people have had and this is not about a choice to just 'drink myself to death.' It's being overwhelmed.
>
> [Substance use professional – focus group]

Further challenges in supporting people who continue to use substances came from visiting family members or friends, for example, visitors who brought substances into the hospice or care setting or were intoxicated when visiting. Therefore, the professionals had to be aware of both the individual's substance use, and any use by their family and friends. They needed to clarify what substance use was acceptable within the hospice (alcohol) and what was not (illicit drugs), as well as the potential dangers of mixing prescribed, licit and illicit substances. Managing someone's care could become more demanding of professionals' time and attention where there were substances involved that complicated medical and social care on the one hand, but also caused stress and concern for the professionals administering that care.

Some professionals had found solutions to some of the challenging scenarios. Two hospices had introduced a system of agreeing who would prescribe the medication – be that the GP, psychiatrist, consultant – essentially one professional only. Another said that good communication between professionals was important, as was communication with the individual themselves:

> … I suppose it's communication and bridging a gap really and trying to explain.
>
> [Hospice professional – focus group]

> Just by being very explicit with people and saying, "This is what this is for and again we expect you to use it in this way, account for every vial of it." We haven't had any vials lost or not accounted for.
>
> [Hospice professional – interviewee]

These practice responses to caring for people who continue to use substances overlap with the challenge of pain and symptom management for people with current or past substance use. These two challenges begin to demonstrate some of the complexity in delivering care in a skilled and informed way and highlighted the current 'trial and error' approach that many staff were taking in the absence of practice guidance and focussed organisational policy.

Discussion and implications

This research was preceded by an awareness of health inequalities faced by people who use substances, but the extent to which those health inequalities impacted access to palliative and end-of-life care were unknown. This research opened a window into the professionals' responses when trying to support people in their care who used substances and were at, or near, the end of their lives. The hospice professionals in particular recounted their own challenges of pain and symptom management for people using substances, and the ignorance they shared with allied professionals about how to respond appropriately when prescribing or administering pain and symptom relief. They shared their fears of both overdosing and under-dosing people – fears that challenged the very purpose of their roles of maximising comfort and minimising pain.

However, this research also found great care and practice with innovative responses and effective cross sector collaborations. The commitment of these professionals to caring for people when they did not want to stop using substances was clear, albeit frustrating and distressing, particularly when the people died. It showed how good palliative care for people using substances was developed from the 'bottom up' and located from a starting position that did not judge or patronise the person. It was also a position that was clear and transparent and did not avoid communicating the, sometimes, unpalatable truth about the implications of continued substance use. Importantly, this was done without moralising or judgement. This was further supplemented with advocacy and empathy when social and health care practitioners failed to deliver appropriate care.

At an individual level, one example of resourcefulness from this research was a nurse administering a small 'tot' of Bourbon to a person in a nursing home with limited vocabulary who was highly agitated and anxious. It worked almost instantly but no one had previously considered that he was possibly withdrawing from ongoing alcohol use – as opposed to just wanting a drink. Yet the nurse who used her initiative feared being criticised for her actions and felt she had broken some professional code when, in fact, her response was proportionate and appropriate. The challenge such individual innovation faces is ensuring there is peer and management support for staff taking initiatives of this kind. This, in turn, will require managers who are informed and knowledgeable about substance use at the end of life.

The professionals also identified the need for further training to develop their confidence in asking about either substance use or the person's wishes for their end of life. While formal training through employment or education is one avenue, there are an increasing number of examples of people taking the initiative and reaching out to local colleagues to join together to learn and collaborate. One example of this is found in the City of Liverpool in the UK where professionals from

Table 3.1 Implications for practice and policy

Implication	How does this involve practitioners?
Develop effective partnership working protocols between substance use and palliative/end-of-life care agencies to support both sets of staff in responding to challenges as they arise.	While this should be developed and embedded at an organisational level, many individual practitioners initiated the good practice we heard about in our research.
Offer local training and practice guidance at an individual staff and organisational level about working with these overlapping issues.	Consider what training you might need and what training you could offer other organisations – by way of a training exchange.
Target local primary and acute health services to build relationships and offer information, training and support.	Use your networks and professional relationships to develop this exchange of expertise. Take the initiative.
Develop practice guidance on pain and symptom management for people with current or previous use of substances at end of life.	There is some early guidance available; see how it fits your work context and adapt it to meet your needs (Action on Addiction, 2013; Quinlan and Cox, 2017).
Ensure support and supervision for staff identifies and addresses the emotional impact of work in this area.	Don't be afraid to ask for emotional support and to flag up to colleagues and managers the impact of this work on your own physical and mental health. Taking care of yourself allows you to take care of others. Model good practice in promoting positive emotional and mental health.
Reviewing training policies to ensure there is a rolling programme of training on substance use and end-of-life care.	Request training on palliative/end-of-life care and substance use; add to training programme including working with significant others too; plan the frequency of rolling programme and book dates; 'sell' the idea to colleagues.
Allocating a policy lead for the development of organisational policy on prescribing, pain and symptom management and its dissemination.	This may be an existing position/person leading on the policy or a new person to take on the lead for this specific project. Develop liaison with policy leads in partner organisations to save work and time.
Developing organisational policy on access to services for this group of people, including issues of routine questioning, appropriate responses, joint working and referral practice, recording and monitoring – to name a few.	Ask for greater support organisationally for work in this area; offer to be part of working group to develop resources and adapt good practice for your agency's needs; reach out to other agencies within your own area of specialism and the 'other' specialism/s to work with you or offer mutual guidance.
Contributing to national-level policy debates around end-of-life care and substance use, particularly with a focus on health inequalities and access to services.	Feedback to managers the gap in knowledge and confidence on this topic; if in leadership position, ensure substance use and end-of-life care are on the agenda at national fora, particularly in response to revisions or developments relating to the Ambitions Framework in palliative and end-of-life care (National Palliative and End of Life Care Partnership, 2021) and debates about 'recovery' focussed substance use services.

a mixed group of disciplinary backgrounds came together to specifically help each other address their shared concerns about people using substances dying in higher numbers and without adequate palliative and end-of-life care. This resulted in a training exchange, improved networking, increased understanding of each other's challenges and an agenda for action. Another is the work of a Canadian group in Vancouver who worked across disciplines and across countries collating evidence to develop a guide for hospital staff for working with "structurally vulnerable patients" including those who use substances (Antifaeff and Robinson, 2021).

Implications for practice and policy

The following implications for practice and policy focus on the themes of this chapter (Table 3.1. Wider implications from the research with the professionals can be found in the full reports and executive summaries (Galvani et al., 2018a, 2018b; Templeton et al., 2018a, 2018b).

Conclusion

Two overlapping themes have been at the core of this chapter: (i) pain and symptom management for people who use (or used to use) substances and are approaching the end of their life, and (ii) care for people who want to continue to use substances as their health deteriorates. What is evident from this research is the extent to which improved knowledge and understanding about these overlapping issues would negate some of the worries that professionals feel. Training and policy development are just two of the complimentary options for furthering such knowledge and understanding. The professionals who participated in this research were finding their own way through these issues when they arose. That is not tenable in the longer term. Fear, frustration or unprocessed loss are not happy bedfellows with safe and effective practice. They are likely to lead to anxiety and potential burnout if left unaddressed. The current evidence suggests we will be seeing more people in services with these overlapping issues. Professionals need to be ready to respond wherever people enter the support system. It is vital that their pre- and post-qualifying education prepares them appropriately for practice. In doing so, it affords them the opportunity to provide the good quality palliative and end-of-life care that they want to offer and that people who use substances deserve.

Key resources

- *Good Practice Guidance: Supporting people with substance problems at the end of life* (Galvani et al., 2019) https://endoflifecaresubstanceuse.com/wp-content/uploads/2022/02/Good-practice-guidance-EoLC-and-SU-April-2019-Web-version.pdf
- *Policy Standards: A Working Document. Palliative and end of life care for people with alcohol and drug problems* (Galvani and Wright, 2019). https://endoflife

caresubstanceuse.com/wp-content/uploads/2022/02/Policy-Standards-SU-and-EoLC-May-2019.pdf
* *Homelessness Palliative Care Toolkit* – http://www.homelesspalliativecare.com/overview-and-faqs/

References

Action on Addiction. (2013) 'The Management of Pain in People with a Past or Current History of Addiction.' Available online at: https://idhdp.com/mediaimport/38281/130607_pain_management_report__final_embargoed_13_june.pdf [Accessed 29th July 2021].

Antifaeff, K., and Robinson, W. (2021) *A Guide for Serious Illness Conversations with Structurally Vulnerable Patients in Hospital.* Vancouver, CA. Available online at: https://www.providencehealthcare.org/sites/default/files/GUIDE_SERIOUS_ILLNESS_CONVERSATIONS_WITH_STRUCTURALLY_VULNERABLE_PATIENTS_IN_HOSPITAL_(V1a).pdf

Ashby, J., Wright, S., and Galvani, S. (2018) *Interviews with People at the End of Life: End of Life Care for People with Alcohol and Drug Problems.* Available online at: https://endoflifecaresubstanceuse.files.wordpress.com/2018/11/end-of-life-care-for-people-with-substance-use-pwe-full-report-final.pdf [Accessed 3rd July 2020].

Brooks, J., and King, N. (2014) *Doing Template Analysis: Evaluating an End of Life Care Service.* Sage Research Methods Cases. DOI: 10.4135/978144627305013512755. Available online at: http://eprints.hud.ac.uk/id/eprint/19707/1/Brooks_and_King_doingTA_EoLCservice.pdf [Accessed 27th July 2018].

Chou, R., Fanciullo, G. J., Fine, P. G., Passik, S. D., and Portenoy, R. K. (2009) 'Opioids for Chronic Noncancer Pain: Prediction and Identification of Aberrant Drug-Related Behaviors: A Review of the Evidence for an American Pain Society and American Academy of Pain Medicine Clinical Practice Guideline.' *The Journal of Pain*, 10(2), pp. 131–146. DOI: 10.1016/j.jpain.2008.10.009

Doukas, N. (2014) 'Are Methadone Counselors Properly Equipped to Meet the Palliative Care Needs of Older Adults in Methadone Maintenance Treatment? Implications for Training.' *Journal of Social Work and End of Life Palliative Care*, 10(2), pp. 186–204. DOI: 10.1080/15524256.2014.906370

Galvani, S. (2018) *End of Life Care for People with Alcohol and Other Drug Problems: What We Know and What We Need To Know. Final Project Report.* Available online at: http://e-space.mmu.ac.uk/622052/1/EOLC%20Final%20overview%20report%2027%20November%202018%20PRINT%20VERSION.pdf [Accessed 4th April 2019].

Galvani, S., Dance, C., and Wright, S. (2018a) *Research Report, Experiences of Hospice and Substance use professionals: End of Life for people with alcohol and Drug Problems.* Manchester: Manchester Metropolitan University. Available online at: https://endoflifecaresubstanceuse.com/wp-content/uploads/2018/11/end-of-life-care-for-people-with-substance-use-professionals-perspective-full-report.pdf

Galvani, S., Dance, C., and Wright, S. (2018b) *Research Briefing No. 5. Experiences of Hospice and Substance use professionals: End of Life for people with alcohol and Drug Problems.* Manchester: Manchester Metropolitan University. Available online at: https://endoflifecaresubstanceuse.com/wp-content/uploads/2018/09/professionals20briefing20final2028th20august202018.pdf

Galvani, S., and Wright, S. (2019) *Supporting People with Substance Problems at the End of Life. Palliative and End of Life Care for People with Alcohol and Drug Problems* (Policy

Standards). Manchester: Manchester Metropolitan University. Available online at: https://endoflifecaresubstanceuse.files.wordpress.com/2019/05/policy-standards-su-and-eolc-may-2019.pdf [Accessed 2nd August 2021].

Galvani, S., Wright, S., and Witham, G. (2019) *Supporting People with Substance Problems at End of Life (Good Practice Guidance)*. Manchester: Manchester Metropolitan University. Available online at: https://endoflifecaresubstanceuse.com/wp-content/uploads/2022/02/Good-practice-guidance-EoLC-and-SU-April-2019-Web-version.pdf [Accessed 22nd March 2022].

Krashin, D., Murinova, N., and Ballantyne, J. (2012) 'Management of Pain with Comorbid Substance Abuse.' *Current Psychiatry Reports*, 14(5), pp. 462–468. DOI: 10.1007/s11920-012-0298-3

Kutzen, H. S. (2004) 'Integration of Palliative Care into Primary Care for Human Immunodeficiency Virus-Infected Patients.' *American Journal of the Medical Sciences*, 328(1), pp. 37–47. DOI: 10.1097/00000441-200407000-00006

Kwon, J. H., Tanco, K., Park, J. C., Wong, A., Seo, L., Liu, D., Chisholm, G., Williams, J., Hui, D., and Bruera, E. (2015) 'Frequency, Predictors, and Medical Record Documentation of Chemical Coping Among Advanced Cancer Patients.' *Oncologist*, 20(6), pp. 692–697. DOI: 10.1634/theoncologist.2015-0012

MacWilliams, J., Bramwell, M., Brown, S., and O'Connor, M. (2014) 'Reaching Out to Ray: Delivering Palliative Care Services to a Homeless Person in Melbourne, Australia.' *International Journal of Palliative Nursing*, 20(2), pp. 83–88. DOI: 10.12968/ijpn.2014.20.2.83

McNeil, R., and Guirguis-Younger, M. (2012) 'Harm Reduction and Palliative Care: Is There a Role for Supervised Drug Consumption Services?' *Journal of Palliative Care*, 28(3), pp. 175–177. DOI: 10.1177/082585971202800308

Morgan, B., & Kochan, K. A. (2008). I'll Always Want More: Complex Issues in HIV Palliative Care. *Journal of Hospice & Palliative Nursing*, 10(5) 265–271. https://doi.org/10.1097/01.NJH.0000319176.48165.44

National Palliative and End of Life Care Partnership. (2021) *Ambitions for Palliative and End of Life Care: A National Framework for Local Action 2021–2026*. Available online at: https://www.england.nhs.uk/blog/renewing-our-ambitions-for-palliative-and-end-of-life-care/ [Accessed 2nd August 2021].

Pancari, J., and Baird, C. (2014) 'Managing Prescription Drug Diversion Risks.' Journal of *Addictions Nursing*, 25(3), pp. 114–121. DOI: 10.1097/JAN.0000000000000036

Passik, S. D., Dhingra, L. K., and Kirsh, K. L. (2009) 'Cancer Pain Management in the Chemically Dependent Patient.' *Cancer Pain: Assessment and Management*, Second Edition, pp. 423–432. DOI: 10.1017/CBO9780511642357.023

Quinlan, J., and Cox, F. (2017) 'Acute Pain Management in Patients with Drug Dependence Syndrome.' *Pain Reports*, 2(4), p. e611. DOI: 10.1097/PR9.0000000000000611. Available online at: https://journals.lww.com/painrpts/fulltext/2017/08000/acute_pain_management_in_patients_with_drug.10.aspx [Accessed 2nd August 2021].

Tan, P. D., Barclay, J. S., and Blackhall, L. J. (2015) 'Do Palliative Care Clinics Screen for Substance Abuse and Diversion? Results of a National Survey.' *Journal of Palliative Medicine*, 18(9), pp. 752–757. DOI: 10.1089/jpm.2015.0098

Taveros, M. C., and Chuang, E. J. (2016) 'Pain Management Strategies for Patients on Methadone Maintenance Therapy: A Systematic Review of the Literature.' *BMJ Supportive and Palliative Care*, 7(4), pp. 383–389. DOI: 10.1136/bmjspcare-2016-001126

Witham, G., Peacock, M., and Galvani, S. (2019) 'End of Life Care for People with Alcohol and Drug Problems: Findings from a Rapid Evidence Assessment.' *Health and Social Care in the Community*, 27(5), pp. e637–e650. DOI: 10.1111/hsc.12807

Yarwood, G. A., Wright, S., Templeton, L., and Galvani, S. (2018). 'End of Life Care for People with Alcohol and Other Drug Problems: Qualitative Analysis of Primary Interviews with Family Members, Friends and Carers.' Available online at: https://endoflifecaresubstanceuse.files.wordpress.com/2018/11/end-of-life-care-for-people-with-substance-use-family-report-phase-2-final-full-report.pdf [Accessed 18th August 2020].

4 Seeing the common ground

Family and practitioner caregivers' perspectives of palliative care for people using substances

Sam Wright, Sarah Galvani and Gemma A. Yarwood

Introduction

This chapter examines caregiving similarities and tensions between families and friends[1] supporting someone who uses substances[2] and has palliative care[3] needs and health and social care practitioners. People who use substances and are approaching the end of life tend to present late to healthcare services (Ashby et al., 2018) resulting in family and friends providing the caregiving role. Typically, the person's health trajectory is unpredictable due to multiple health conditions. They may not recognise the full extent of their symptoms, partly because their substance use can mask how ill they are. They may also be reluctant to engage with services. This means that they, their family carers, and the health and social care practitioners working with them, have very little time to forge the working relationships that will help them to achieve a dignified death.

Palliative care research and practice recognise the importance of families and practitioners communicating effectively to bring about good end-of-life care, while also acknowledging the challenges of working together (Leadership Alliance for the Care of Dying People, 2014; National Palliative and End-of-life care Partnership, 2015; Standing et al., 2020; Virdun et al., 2015). Substance use adds yet more complications, not least the long-term impact of the emotional strain that many family members experience when living with, or caring for, someone using substances, including the prospect that their loved one will die unexpectedly or prematurely (Valentine et al., 2018; Yarwood et al., 2018). The strain family members face is mirrored in the heightened levels of practitioner concern over potential challenging behaviours from both the person using substances and/or their substance using friends and family (Galvani et al., 2018). This already complex combination of factors can be further exacerbated by professional uncertainty about how to treat someone using substances at the end of life.

Reflecting silos in policy, practice and academic enquiry (Galvani, 2018; Galvani et al., 2019), research typically focusses on *either* substance use or palliative care. However, combining knowledge about substance use and palliative care is at the heart of our research and provided inspiration for this book. In developing this chapter, and in conversations between ourselves as authors, we realised that addressing family experiences singularly would articulate only one side of the

DOI: 10.4324/9781003187882-5

story and risked alienating practitioners by ignoring their viewpoints. Our aim therefore is to uncover the 'middle ground' where the shared priorities of families and practitioners caring for someone with both substance use and palliative care support needs can be explored. Hopefully this is one step towards promoting more compassionate understanding and, as a result, greater collaborative care.

In this chapter, we draw on qualitative data from three strands of our mixed methods end-of-life care and substance use study (Galvani, 2018) to discuss how differing perspectives can compromise care. We explore how poor (or absent) communication can lead to polarised perspectives between practitioners and family members and provide some insights into the common ground between them to offer a more helpful reconstruction of that 'social reality'. By unpicking the separate standpoints between families and practitioners in this way, we offer an alternative framing to show how differing priorities and needs can be better conjoined.

The study and participants

Like the rest of this section, this chapter draws on data from a programme of research designed to consolidate and extend the limited existing knowledge about end-of-life care for people using substances (Galvani, 2018). This chapter presents findings from three qualitative strands of the study which comprised interviews with:

i   Eighteen family members currently or previously providing care for relatives who used substances and were approaching the end of their lives;
ii Fifty-three health and social care practitioners working in hospices or substance use teams; and
iii Twenty key informants (policy makers and practitioners working in this specialised field).

Interviews with family caregivers sought to explore both how they experienced their relative's end of life, and the extent to which services recognised or responded to the whole family's needs. The interviews with practitioners and key informants also sought to elicit examples of good practice as well as the challenges faced when caring for people with both support needs.

Box 4.1 Note for future research

It is important to note that whilst our research gathered experiences from practitioners working in hospices and substance use teams, most of the families' criticisms of care were based on their experiences of primary and acute care. This is an area for future research and practice improvement

---

The emotional strain of caring for people using substances at end of life

For many families where a relative has a life-shortening condition, relationships may be under strain both before diagnosis and during their subsequent care, challenging simplistic notions of family as a mutually sustaining and supportive environment (Monroe and Oliviere, 2008). But where the person who is dying also uses substances, this stress is likely to add to years of prior emotional strain, including anticipatory grief (over loss of intimacy with their relative), as well as anxiety over their possible premature death (Da Silve et al., 2007; Oreo and Ozgul, 2007). Many of the family interviewees described years of offering extensive care and support in response to their relative's substance use:

> It's been horrific for everyone involved. For all of us...it's 14 years of daily care, which is a massive impact on everyone.... I haven't been on holiday for ten years, I don't think my mum's been for like 16 or something. So it's very hard. It affects everyone... Basically, me and my mum were his carers for the last 14 years and it's not financially viable. It makes you very depressed sometimes. It's very tiring. It's a big responsibility and I don't think you should have to deal with [it alone].
>
> Sister, Brother died alone at home

While each family had a unique history, they commonly described the enormous impact, stress and multiple disadvantages that they had experienced over a prolonged period of time caring for a relative who used substances. This caused direct and indirect harm to their well-being as individuals and families. Some practitioners acknowledged this emotional toll, discussing the years of strain and care prior to the palliative care diagnosis:

> The family that are around will have had ... a bad time with them [the dying relative] over the years and quite often – through guilt – will continue to look after them. But will have been treated quite badly.
>
> Key Informant, Frontline HSCP

Understandably, family members could feel extremely frustrated and distressed that their relative was dying, particularly if there was a direct link between their substance use and their premature death. Many practitioners understood and empathised with the longstanding emotional difficulties families were undergoing:

> When you speak to those families, families themselves can get angry, because they feel that this person has done it to themselves.
>
> Hospice professional – focus group

Some health and social care practitioners we interviewed were aware of the support needs of family members – even though they were not in a position to provide it:

> There is a massive need for them to get psychological support, to actually deal with it…there's limited availability in the area, we don't have … psychological support. So it's us who supports them to look after [their relative] and it can be very difficult because there's two needy people there who are needing access to support.
>
> Frontline health and social care practitioner

However, practitioners also felt the emotional strain even among those who knew the person was very ill or dying:

> For all of us, somebody dying, we're at risk of feeling a bit of a failure really and I'm not sure that we've totally yet got to the way of looking at how we can think about a good death. … When you're in a generic service and somebody dies, you think, "Oh my God." Either: "What could we have done better?" Or: "If only he'd stopped drinking." … I don't think that there's a lot of preparation as staff that we have for these situations. Let alone supporting a client who's in this predicament.
>
> Substance use professional – interviewee

> The biggest thing … I'm trying to learn [is that] things aren't always…, you can't always totally resolve [patients' problems] in the end.
>
> Hospice professional – focus group

While different for each individual, this emotional impact when a person dies is one area of mutual experience between family and practitioner caregivers:

Poor communication of palliative care need

For many family members, it had taken a number of years, multiple symptoms and numerous GP or hospital appointments before the severity of their loved one's

---

Box 4.2 Common ground 1

Common ground 1: While the sense of loss is often greater among family members, there is nevertheless a shared experience of sadness between family and practitioners when the person they care for dies. This is often accompanied by some self-questioning of whether more could have been done to delay death – meaning that both family and practitioners would benefit from emotional support and an opportunity to air their frustrations and anxieties.

condition was recognised. Even then, medical professionals often had not explicitly communicated that their relative was approaching the end of their life:

> We got to a point where he did start to deteriorate and we noticed he was [be] coming ill…nothing was diagnosed for sure…and then we noticed the yellowing of his skin and his eyes and this was where he kept saying, 'I feel so terrible.'
> Nephew, Uncle died in hospital

Lack of explicit identification of a life-shortening health condition meant that relatives were rarely able to access palliative care and the family members' own support needs were usually unacknowledged. Among the people participating in our research, referral to palliative care was rare. One example was a young man (the brother of the interviewee), who had stage four kidney failure and was on the transplant list. Not only was his health deteriorating, but his situation was clearly complex: he had learning difficulties, was not managing his diabetes well, had chronic pain, was experiencing depression and also using substances:

> We weren't signposted to anything decent. I'm going to say it's a very niche thing, but there must be so many people suffering from the same type of things in this area. Sister, Brother died alone at home.

Aside from the historical frustration and strained relationships that can exist within families where a member uses substances, there can be distressing physical and mental health symptoms as the person's health deteriorates. Practitioners were conflicted over the extent to which they should explicitly warn families about potential symptoms or manifestations of their relative's illness, wanting to prepare them for distressing situations, while not exacerbating their anxiety over what their loved one might face. Getting the balance right will inevitably be a difficult task. However, it is important that practitioners at least start conversations with family members about the challenges that a substance-related death may entail, sensitively recognising the added complexity and that distress it can bring for family.

The need for family members to have a clear diagnosis – even if that includes uncertainty over the prognosis – is clear. Specialist palliative care practitioners could help families by supporting effective communication between them and their relative about their illness and their wishes for the end of their lives. They could also speak to the family about what palliative care can offer, and how the person's substance use may or may not influence the care provided.

Substance use practitioners faced similar challenges in understanding someone's diagnosis and prognosis. They spoke of the fluctuating condition of someone's health that mimicked, and was exacerbated by, their changing patterns of substance use. It made 'predicting' end of life and tailoring care accordingly, particularly difficult:

> …the cancer things are quite predictable, you can almost see where things are. But with the organic deaths, it's this lumpy bumpy graph that you don't know where you are from one minute to the next…
> Substance use practitioner focus group

Once client permission to share information is given, practitioners can find family members' insights to be helpful in determining the person's health status and planning for their care:

> …because you're going to have clients that obviously sit down and go, "Yeah, yeah I'm fine. I'm fine. Yeah, nothing wrong with me, I'm fine." And then, when you talk to the family members they'll say, "Well, actually they had a really bad week last week and they was really down." And then you can talk to them again the next time you see them.
>
> Substance use professional – interviewee

Overcoming stereotypes and challenging stigma

Unfortunately, many people's previous attempts to access primary and acute health services – either as someone using substances or as their family carer – were often poor, featuring experiences of being stigmatised and dismissed. This led to a quite natural wariness towards services. One female ex-partner described how her previous experiences of discrimination (when she had been a drug user) and negative interactions with a range of health and social care practitioners had left her mistrustful of services following her ex-partner's death. She reflects on whether, in hindsight, trying to explain more about their drug using histories might have brought about a more understanding response from the health practitioners:

> Maybe I should have tried to get them [district nurses] to understand. But I think for me, my barriers were coming up more and more and because – I think it's like anything: if somebody starts to attack you, I don't so much usually attack back, now I just tend to go: "Oh fuck you." And put barriers up and just carry on as best as possible. But I do agree, maybe if I had explained more of, "It's really difficult because emotionally we haven't grown up and we struggle with our emotions." That probably would have made a big difference. But I do think as addicts, we get so pissed off having to explain ourselves.
>
> Female ex-partner, Former partner died at home

Box 4.3　Common ground 2

Common ground 2: The combination of substance use and complex health conditions can make prognosis unpredictable but both practitioners and families need clear communication to facilitate their role in caregiving. Practitioners have a delicate balancing act of trying to share helpful information while not overloading the family with distressing details. This necessitates building rapport from an early stage – to allow everyone to work towards a good and dignified death.

This sense that she should perhaps have 'explained more' reveals how communication barriers between practitioners and families can cause substantial difficulties: solidifying resentments about stigmatised identities and past negative service experiences.

Negative stereotypes about people 'addicted' to substances can also influence perceptions of their families and close friends, with outsiders assuming that they are implicated in, or to blame for, their relative's substance use (Guy, 2004; Guy and Holloway, 2007; Chapple et al., 2015). Many families had experienced social isolation and an associated lack of support because of their relative's substance use. Sadly, several of them reported prejudiced attitudes from some health practitioners within primary and acute healthcare settings – resulting in both poor treatment for their relative and an absence of emotional support for them. For example, at one point when the family of a man dying from liver failure suggested to hospital staff that their loved one needed to be in a hospice, the response they received was: 'There's nothing we can do about that'. One of the family members was later told by a nurse to provide personal care to their loved one themselves, because staff were too busy. He told us:

> I changed the bed and I bagged everything up, I got these wipes and [the nurse] said, 'If you're going to make [the bed], at least make it properly.' And I said: 'It's not my fucking job'.
>
> Nephew, Uncle died in hospital

This family's experience reveals how negative practitioner attitudes towards people who use substances can 'spill over' into deprioritising their care and actual neglect: revealing how crucial it is to provide staff with training and challenge any discriminatory beliefs (Galvani and Wright, 2019). The family also highlighted the importance of compassionate approaches to supporting carers:

> Why did they always have a stern, cold exterior to everything that they said? Whenever you spoke to them, it was so abrupt and there was no feeling. There was nothing there… they should at least empathise with the family.
>
> Nephew, Uncle died in hospital

While any family could have experienced poor, uncompassionate professional care, interviewees believed that their experiences had been based in negative practitioner judgements about their relative's substance use. Another research participant described how carers coming into her ex-partner's house in the last months of his life were overly suspicious, expecting a high-risk environment:

> It's not like they were walking to a house with needles all over the floor; or we were threatening them or smashed out of our faces. I wasn't using anymore. Even when I was using, I wasn't like that. I still had a really clean house, lived in a completely normal life.
>
> Female ex-partner, Partner died at home

Some family members had realised that they needed to instil boundaries to the care they provided – to prevent the emotional burden they were facing from damaging their own well-being. Unfortunately, this could lead to practitioners misinterpreting these emotional boundaries as suggesting an uncaring or neglectful attitude from them. One interviewee described her feeling of being stigmatised by a nurse who was judgemental of her limiting her contact with her father – a decision she felt she had to take to protect her own mental health. Similarly, this son felt judged initially by nursing staff when he was finally able to persuade his father to attend hospital:

> We took him to hospital and because of the state that he was in….they took photographs of his legs…I also was a little bit, well, quite angry because there was some suggestion that I had completely neglected him. That I had just left him there to rot at home…I understand it on a very basic level. But obviously they didn't know the history… it's also very important to establish all the facts and the situation before laying blame as it were.
>
> Son, Father died in hospital

There were, in counterbalance, numerous examples of good care – typically from hospices and substance use services. One family was particularly effusive in their praise of a peer volunteer from an alcohol service who had supported them:

> [The alcohol service] are the only people that have been an absolute rock to this family since [relative's] passing. [Volunteer], I couldn't thank him enough. I will be eternally grateful to [volunteer] for what he's done…from the word go when they first come here, they put themselves out that much to do things for [relative] and us. They took us both in like family and helped us right the way through… they've provided aftercare to the family that have been bereaved and they need to be recognised for that. Family, Relative died in hospital

Providing palliative care when family carers use substances

It is important to be realistic in recognising that, in their role as informal carers, all families have the potential to either help professional care by supporting their

---

Box 4.4 Common ground 3

Common ground 3: A greater mutual understanding of the stress and strain of the caregiving role on the family members might lessen judgemental attitudes. This can be achieved through empathetic and compassionate care, active listening skills and explicit acknowledgement of the anger, pain and need for psychological support that often accompanies caring for people who use substances.

relative effectively or, conversely, negatively impact both their relative and the practitioners working with them. This is why practitioners need the knowledge and skills to be able to forge good, trusting relationships with families whenever possible.

Practitioners in our research spoke of the challenges that substance using family members presented to the care of their relative. Practitioners shared their concerns about how family carers who used substances might impede delivery of a patient's palliative care, particularly in the home. From a hospice perspective, there were concerns about the safety of take-home prescription medicines for people approaching end of life when other people who used substances lived, or had access to, their home. Concerns related not just to the diversion of drugs into the community, but also the safety of everyone in the home if substance use was not managed carefully. One hospice practitioner related the story of a young intravenous drug user living with an elderly person, where neither were coping with the situation:

> So, the police come. Then an ambulance comes. And I've had to literally back out and do like an incident to Social Services for safeguarding. They came back, and actually he'd been putting dirty needles in his father's commode and one of the ambulance men that were moving him nearly got a needlestick [injury].
>
> Hospice professional – focus group

Other challenges included family members bringing substances into the relative's home or hospice or being intoxicated themselves. Practitioners spoke of the medical risks posed for the person in their care, putting them in the position of needing to 'challenge' the family members – arguably not the best basis upon which to build good relationships. Indeed, some hospice staff working in peoples' homes were concerned about the aggression they could face from family members who were using substances. Hospice staff talked about the difficult ethical position they faced when working in homes where illicit substances were used: questioning what they could do and how far they could 'step in' to raise the issue with the family members concerned. A hospice community nurse visiting someone at home described how they had explained to a family about the need to stop people visiting who were providing illicit drugs to their dying relative, as it negated the care they provided:

> It was also [about] speaking to the family and saying: "Look, if you know who these people are, you need to speak to them and stop them from coming because this is not helping him and it doesn't help us."
>
> Hospice professional – focus group

Practitioners wanted people to be open about the potential for medications to be stolen, so that appropriate measures could be put in place. Those safety measures might include the use of a lock box or arrangements between social and health care practitioners for only one prescriber rather than several from different services. There was also concern about the management of 'stockpiled' drugs that people no longer needed – a particular concern was that family members who used substances might be tempted to use the medications prescribed for their relative as a coping mechanism in their bereavement. There was, however, a reflection that many nurses' fears about risks related to drug use may be disproportionate – potentially leading them to put a lock box in place even if a family member had not used drugs for many years and currently lived hundreds of miles away.

Relatives visiting hospices in an intoxicated state could also be challenging for staff. In one focus group, participants described having to put intoxicated relatives into a taxi to make their way home.

Other examples of challenges from family members included:

- Causing disruption in hospital and being physically and verbally aggressive towards staff
- Disagreement within families and with hospital staff about their loved one's care
- Airing views that the person had brought their problems on themselves
- Wanting the focus to be on them and their suffering
- Blaming professionals for their loved one's condition and death.

Post-death – the need for specialist support

The provision of ongoing support for bereaved families is important. It can be particularly difficult for families if a death has to be referred for a post-mortem examination or to a coroner (Galvani et al., 2018; Valentine 2017). At such times, the family may be anxious that they have done something wrong or that someone has either overprescribed or administered too much medication. Police involvement only further escalates tensions and anxieties.

The frustration and anger families often feel about a relative's substance use during their lives is often accompanied by shame and stigma for family members too. This can continue post-death, taking a particularly destructive toll on family members (Chapple et al., 2015), partly because of the premature and often

---

Box 4.5 Common ground 4

Common ground 4: Family members who use substances are not all the same and are likely to need support in their own right. Some of them will facilitate good care, others may hinder it (unintentionally or otherwise). Accepting that both family and professional caregivers can help or hinder the care each other provides could help to build a stronger mutual sense of interdependence. Equally importantly, this will keep the best interests of the person at end of life at the heart of the care plan.

avoidable nature of the death (Da Silve et al., 2007; Degenhardt et al., 2014; Nambiar et al., 2015). Feelings of shame, guilt and stigma heighten the pain of bereavement (Feigelman et al., 2011; Chapple et al., 2015). Therefore, it is not surprising that some practitioners had encountered families who were very reluctant for their loved one's alcohol or drug use to be named as the cause of death on their death certificate:

> Families do not like alcoholic liver disease, so they do not want that putting on the death certificate. So there's pressure on doctors who've got a family that's recently bereaved.
>
> KI interviewee – Other Professional

In summary, our data revealed both positive and negative relationships between social and health care practitioners and family members. Both groups have such an important role to play in supporting people to have the best death possible, but where substance use is part of the picture, suspicion and distrust looms large for both parties. Substance use within the family can undermine professional care and pose risks to staff safety. Yet practitioners need to not operate on the mistrustful assumptions that focus solely on risk-avoidance and are communicated defensively.

Discussion

While families share many experiences and support needs with other groups of carers, they also face unique difficulties (Hudson and Payne, 2008) not least in having to continuously review health and social care needs and make adaptations as their relative's health declines (NCPC, 2012; Payne and EAPC Taskforce, 2010). As such, they may be involved in discussing care priorities with their relative, helping them to make choices, and supporting them to communicate their end-of-life wishes. Other families, perhaps estranged from their relative through choice or circumstance, may not have the capacity to provide palliative or end-of-life care.

Box 4.6 Common ground 5

Common ground 5: Practitioner assumptions about substance use can easily lead to families feeling stigmatised, leaving a legacy of negative feelings about asking for support in the future. A better approach that ensures good care for the person approaching end of life while also supporting both family members and practitioners into bereavement is needed. Effective communication that exudes compassion is the cornerstone to such good palliative practice.

In either case, our research suggests support for family members is limited at best. Poor communication between family members and health and social care practitioners was a key part of the problem, underpinned by perceived and actual negative attitudes from some practitioners. Improving care for both people who use substances and their family carers requires the development of trusting relationships between practitioners and the family. Even those family members who may hinder care may do so without malice. For example, substance use may be a significant part of their life and may be a shared experience with their relative. They may now suddenly feel dislocated and disrupted from their shared normality and routines at the end of life.

Without good formal support, the burden of palliative care places heavy demands on family caregivers, often to the detriment of their own well-being (Wittenberg et al., 2017). Family caregiver support needs can include psychological and emotional needs; their own physical ill health; insufficient symptom management skills; limited respite time; deteriorating family circumstances; financial difficulties and inadequate health or social care input (Hudson, 2004; Payne and European Association for Palliative Care Taskforce, 2010). There is considerable value, therefore, in health and social care practitioners providing timely, tailored support to family carers (Mathieson et al., 2020). An important component of this is provision of the information and skills training necessary to undertake physical nursing tasks (Bee et al., 2009; Connolly and Milligan, 2014). By increasing family carers' mastery of care tasks, as well as their confidence to do them, they are likely to find it easier to accept the practical support that enables them to provide care – although they still may not recognise the extent to which they need emotional help for themselves (Grande et al., 2009).

Yet one substantial constraint is that families and practitioners involved in end-of-life care are often brought together in crisis, with only a short period of time to facilitate a peaceful and dignified death for the person they both care for. For them to work closely together, practitioners and families need to be able to openly communicate their concerns, share knowledge about the person's condition and resolve any challenges. This makes it all the more crucial that practitioners are able to reflect on, and counter, any personal bias they may hold against people who use substances and their social networks. This can be achieved through effective use of supervision, continuing professional development and honest conversation about feelings with peers. There may well be pre-existing, challenging, family dynamics (Young Bushfield and De Ford, 2010), and families may have different patterns of informal social support than those that palliative care practitioners are used to working with. Family relationships will have been constructed and negotiated over many years, whereas the practitioner relationship will be new – bringing external observations and judgements to what is often a sensitive situation. Any negative assumptions can lead families and practitioners separately to perceive themselves 'at odds' with the other party, and to position themselves in opposition to the other. Whereas, if we can encourage both to acknowledge the commonalities between them, they can hopefully recognise what needs to be communicated to each other and work together collaboratively. It is, therefore, imperative that families and practitioners cooperate to break down pre-existing assumptions and pave the way to more effective communication and compassionate care.

Figure 4.1 offers a simple summary of the positions that health and social care practitioners and families may take if operating alone – as well as clarifying the 'middle ground' where families and practitioners share common concerns and goals.

- Shared uncertainty over health prognosis, substance use and related behaviours
- Shared concern about 'doing the wrong thing' and being judged
- Shared desire to provide person with a dignified death and best possible care for them and their families
- Shared sense of loss and need for emotional support after death.

Diagram 1 Common ground between practitioners and family carers

Palliative care at its most beneficial is compassionate, collaborative, coordinated and tailored to individual need. It facilitates the delivery of responsive, needs-led care that supports both the patient and the family in its own right. However, in the absence of open communication from the individual or their family members about the person's substance use, practitioners will struggle to meet their support needs. This can be catastrophic to families: compounding existing family tensions surrounding their relative's substance use as they die, and potentially deepening the trauma of seeing their relative die with little or no formal support (Yarwood et al., 2018). The common ground identified here in the midst of these

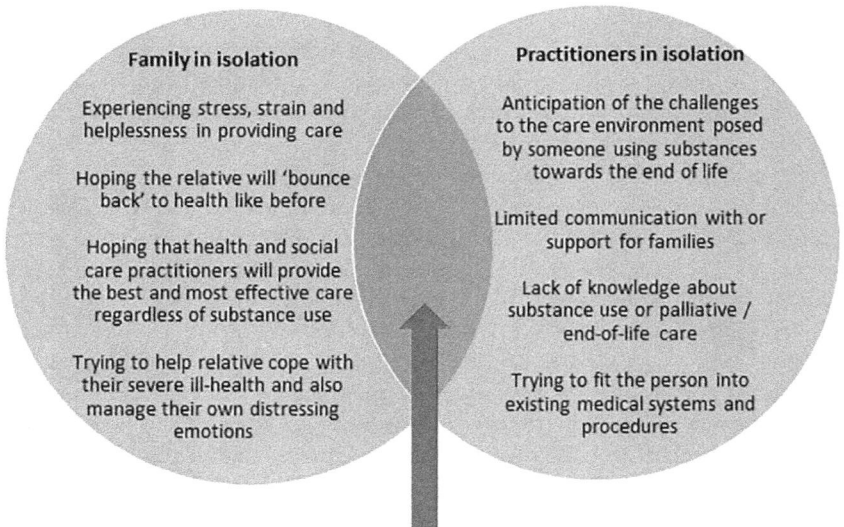

Figure 4.1 Common ground: weaving perspectives together.

complex and constructed perspectives offers a basis on which to develop mutual understanding of, and better support for, family and professional caregivers.

Conclusion

Effective and compassionate communication is the foundation for building mutual understanding of the needs of family members, their dying relative and the practitioners who provide palliative care. Creating good, trusting relationships between informal and professional carers can support the identification and understanding of problems, decision-making and problem-solving. However, it must be done from a non-judgemental position about a person's substance use, and an understanding of the possible feeling of mistrust for services held by people who uses substances and their families. The family and practitioner experiences presented in this chapter provide powerful illustrations of how effective communication and shared values of care need to be at centre of relationships between family and formal caregivers. For practitioners, good communication needs to be shored up by education, training, ongoing support and genuine, mutual respect. For family members, clarity from practitioners about what will help and/or hinder their relative's care, can pave the way to recognising the shared goal of providing the best possible care and most peaceful and dignified death for their relative.

Notes

1 Hereafter 'family'.
2 Including both current and past use of alcohol and other drugs.
3 For the purpose of this chapter, we use palliative care as an umbrella term to include end-of-life care.

References

Ashby, J., Wright, S. and Galvani, S. (2018) *End of life care for people with alcohol and other drug problems: interviews with people with end of life care needs who have substance problems.* Manchester, Manchester Metropolitan University. https://endoflifecaresubstanceuse.com/wp-content/uploads/2018/11/end-of-life-care-for-people-with-substance-use-pwe-full-report-final.pdf [Accessed 21st March 2022].
Bee, P.E., Barnes, P. and Luker, K.A. (2009) 'A systematic review of informal caregivers' needs in providing home-based end-of-life care to people with cancer.' *Journal of Clinical Nursing*, 18(10), pp. 1379–1393. DOI: 10.1111/j.1365-2702.2008.02405.x
Chapple, A., Ziebland, S. and Hawton, K. (2015) 'Taboo and the different death? Perceptions of those bereaved by suicide or other traumatic death.' *Sociology of Health and Illness*, 37, pp. 610–625. DOI: 10.1111/1467-9566.12224
Connolly, J. and Milligan, S. (2014) 'Knowledge and skills needed by informal carers to look after terminally ill patients at home.' *End of Life Journal*, 4(2), pp. 1–14. https://caregiversns.org/images/uploads/all/Knowledge_and_skills_needed_by_informal_carers_to_look_after_terminally_ill_patients_at_home_End_of_Life_Journal.htm_.pdf [Accessed 4th March 2022].

Da Silve, E., Noto, A. and Formigoni, M. (2007) 'Death by drug overdose: impact on families.' *Journal of Psychoactive Drugs*, 39, pp. 301–306. DOI: 10.1080/02791072.2007.10400618

Degenhardt, L., Larney, S., Randall, D., Burns, L. and Hall, W. (2014) 'Causes of death in a cohort treated for opioid dependence between 1985 and 2005.' *Addiction*, 109, pp. 90–99. DOI: 10.1111/add.12337

Feigelman, W., Gorman, B.S. and Jordan, J. (2011) 'Parental grief after a child's drug death compared to other death causes: investigating a greatly neglected bereavement problem population.' *Omega Journal of Death and Dying*, 63, pp. 291–316. DOI: 10.2190/om.63.4.a

Galvani, S. (2018) *End of life care for people with alcohol and other drug problems: what we know and what we need to know*. Final Project Report. Manchester Metropolitan University. Available online at: http://e-space.mmu.ac.uk/622052/1/EOLC%20Final%20overview%20report%2027%20November%202018%20PRINT%20VERSION.pdf [Accessed 4th March 2022].

Galvani, S., Dance, C. and Wright, S. (2018) *End of life care for people with alcohol and other drug problems: report on practitioner experiences of providing care*. Manchester, Manchester Metropolitan University. https://endoflifecaresubstanceuse.com/wp-content/uploads/2018/11/end-of-life-care-for-people-with-substance-use-professionals-perspective-full-report.pdf [Accessed 21st March 2022].

Galvani, S. and Wright, S. (2019) *Supporting people with substance problems at the end of life supporting people with substance problems at the end of life supporting people with substance problems at the end of life supporting people with substance problems at the end of life palliative and end of life care for people with alcohol and drug problems (Policy Standards)*. Manchester, Manchester Metropolitan University. https://endoflifecaresubstanceuse.com/wp-content/uploads/2022/02/Policy-Standards-SU-and-EoLC-May-2019.pdf [Accessed 4th March 2022].

Galvani, S., Wright, S. and Witham, G. (2019) *Supporting people with substance problems at end of life (Good Practice Guidance)*. Manchester, Manchester Metropolitan University. https://endoflifecaresubstanceuse.com/wp-content/uploads/2022/02/Good-practice-guidance-EoLC-and-SU-April-2019-Web-version.pdf [Accessed 4th March 2022].

Grande, G., Stajduhar, K. Aoun, S., Toye, C., Funk, L., Addington-Hall, J., Payne, S. and Todd, C. (2009) 'Supporting lay carers in end of life care: current gaps and future priorities.' *Palliative Medicine*, 23(4), pp. 339–344. Epub 2009 Mar 20. PMID: 19304804. DOI: 10.1177/0269216309104875

Guy, P. (2004) 'Bereavement through drug use: messages from research.' *Practice*, 16, pp. 43–54. DOI: 10.1080/0950315042000254956

Guy, P. and Holloway, M. (2007) 'Drug-related deaths and the 'special deaths' of late modernity.' *Sociology*, 41, pp. 83–96. DOI: 10.1177/0038038507074717

Hudson, P. (2004) 'Positive aspects and challenges associated with caring for a dying relative at home.' *International Journal of Palliative Nursing*, 10(2), pp. 58–65. DOI: 10.12968/ijpn.2004.10.2.12454

Hudson, P. and Payne, S. (2008) *Family carers in palliative care: a guide for health and social care professionals*. Oxford, Oxford University Press. DOI: 10.1093/acprof:oso/9780199216901.001.0001

Leadership Alliance for the Care of Dying People. (2014) *One chance to get it right: improving people's experience of care in the last few days and hours of life*. Available online at: https://www.gov.uk/government/uploads/system/uploads/attachment_data/file/323188/One_chance_to_get_it_right.pdf [Accessed 27th July 2018].

Mathieson, A., Luker, K. and Grande, G. (2020) '"It's like trying to ice a cake that's not been baked": a qualitative exploration of the contextual factors associated with implementing an evidence-based information intervention for family carers at the end of life.' *Primary Health Care Research and Development*, 21, p. e52. DOI: 10.1017/S146342362000050X

Monroe, B. and Oliviere, D. (2008) 'Communicating with family carers.' In Hudson, P. and Payne, S. (Eds.) *Family carers in palliative care: a guide for health and social care professionals.* Oxford, Oxford University Press. DOI: 10.1093/acprof:oso/9780199216901.003.0001

Nambiar, D., Weir, A., Aspinall, E., Stoove, M., Hutchinson, S., Dietze, P., Waugh, L. and Goldberg, D. (2015) 'Mortality and cause of death in a cohort of people who had ever injected drugs in Glasgow: 1982–2012.' *Drug and Alcohol Dependence*, 147, pp. 215–221. DOI: 10.1016/j.drugalcdep.2014.11.008

National Council for Palliative Care. (NCPC) (2012) *Who cares? Support for carers of people approaching the end of life.* Available online at: http://www.ncpc.org.uk/sites/default/files/Who_Cares_Conference_Report.pdf [Accessed 27th July 2018].

National Palliative and End of Life Care Partnership. (2015) *Ambitions for palliative and end of life care: a national framework for local action 2015–2020.* Available online at: http://endoflifecareambitions.org.uk/wp-content/uploads/2015/09/Ambitions-forPalliative-and-End-of-Life-Care.pdf [Accessed 27th July 2018].

Oreo, A. and Ozgul, S. (2007) 'Grief experiences of parents coping with an adult child with problem substance use.' *Addiction Research and Theory*, 15, pp. 71–83. DOI: 10.1080/16066350601036169

Payne, S. and European Association for Palliative Care Taskforce. (2010) 'EAPC update White Paper on improving support for family carers in palliative care: parts 1 and 2.' *European Journal of Palliative Care* 238, 17(5). Available at: https://www.eapcnet.eu/wp-content/uploads/2021/03/Family-carers-2010.pdf [Accessed 28th February 2022]

Standing, H., Patterson, R., Lee, M., Dalkin, S.M., Lhussier M., Bate, A., Exley C. and Brittain K. (2020) 'Information sharing challenges in end-of-life care: a qualitative study of patient, family and professional perspectives on the potential of an electronic palliative care co-ordination system.' *BMJ Open*, 10, p. e037483. DOI: 10.1136/bmjopen-2020-037483

Valentine, C. (2017) *Families bereaved by alcohol or drugs: research on experiences, coping and support.* London, Routledge. ISBN 9780367178659. DOI: 10.4324/9781315670294

Valentine, C., McKell, J. and Ford, A. (2018) 'Service failures and challenges in responding to people bereaved through drugs and alcohol: An interprofessional analysis.' *Journal of Interprofessional Care*, 32:3, 295–303, DOI: 10.1080/13561820.2017.1415312

Virdun, C., Luckett, T., Davidson, P. and Phillips, J. (2015) 'Dying in the hospital setting: a systematic review of quantitative studies identifying the elements of end-of-life care that patients and their families rank as being most important.' *Palliative Medicine*, 9, pp. 774–796. DOI: 10.1177/0269216315583032

Wittenberg, Y., Kwekkeboom, R., Staaks, J., Verhoeff, A. and de Boer, A. (2017) Informal caregivers' views on the division of responsibilities between themselves and professionals: a scoping review. *Health and Social Care in the Community*, pp. 1–14. DOI: 10.1111/hsc.12529

Yarwood, G., Wright, S., Templeton, L. and Galvani, S. (2018) *End of life care for people with alcohol and other drug problems: qualitative analysis of primary interviews with family members, friends and carers.* Manchester, Manchester Metropolitan University. https://endoflifecaresubstanceuse.com/wp-content/uploads/2018/11/end-of-life-care-for-people-with-substance-use-family-report-phase-2-final-full-report1.pdf [Accessed 21st March 2022].

Young Bushfield, S. and DeFord, B. (2010) *End of life care and addictions: a family systems approach.* New York, Springer. ISBN: 9780826121417. DOI: 10.1080/00981389.2011.603997

Part II

Health inequalities

Introduction by Sarah Galvani

The chapters contained in Part II of this book focus primarily on health inequalities. There is a considerable overlap between health and social inequalities, with one rarely existing without the other, so it is a reluctant separation from Part III. However, the work in Part II seeks to foreground the experiences of four groups of people whose needs, in addition to palliative and end-of-life care and substance use, are seen by services as primarily health focussed; these are people with limited health literacy, people with learning disabilities, those living with mental ill health and people living with hepatitis C. What these chapters have in common is a critique of partnership and collaborative care, part of which is the difficulties of appropriate and meaningful communication based on the person's needs, not the system's needs. They also all report on levels of stigma and discrimination that got in the way of communicating and delivering respectful, appropriate and good care. In Chapter 5, Witham presents the concept of health literacy that is a thread that runs throughout Part II chapters. Without a degree of health literacy, people's access to and understanding of care is likely to fail as they try to navigate a system they little understand and is not sufficiently communicated by practitioners who fail to understand people's needs. In Chapter 6, Witham and Galvani highlight the isolation and stigma people with learning disabilities face through the eyes of Grace. Grace, a sister to Peter who had multiple needs in addition to learning disabilities and substance use, reports how such isolation and stigma is extended even to family members. Grace reports a lack of meaningful engagement with herself and Peter that led to her conclude that Peter's life was not valued by practitioners. Webb, in Chapter 7, shows how discrimination and stigmatisation of people with co-existing mental ill health and substance use leads them to present late to services because of their reluctance to engage with systems that are judgemental and exclusionary. She highlights how cumulative problems combined with trauma leaves people unable to navigate complex care pathways. The final chapter in this section, Chapter 8, explores older people injecting substances with a particular focus on people with hepatitis C conditions. Higgs flags up the "constant negotiation with service providers" that is required to get care, which is particularly difficult for a cohort of people who are often of

DOI: 10.4324/9781003187882-6

limited formal education, living in insecure housing and facing frequent stigma and discrimination. What the chapters in this part call for is a far greater emphasis on meeting the person where they are at – a real needs-led approach, rather than what people currently experience as a systems-led approach.

5 Health literacy and substance use within palliative and end-of-life care

Gary Witham

Introduction

This chapter will explore health literacy and examine its definitions and scope. We will further examine the significance of health literacy and its application to both palliative and end-of-life care in relation to substance use. A more detailed exploration of both health literacy related to people using substances at the end of life and formal/informal carers will be included. We will then examine strategies to support health literacy from a social ecological approach and use a practice example of pain management at the end of life.

Definitions and scope of health literacy

Health literacy is an ill-defined concept and has been explained and redefined historically to address contemporary cultural discourses at that time (Berkman et al., 2010). The World Health Organisation defines health literacy as:

> Health literacy is linked to literacy and entails people's knowledge, motivation and competences to access, understand, appraise and apply health information in order to make judgements and take decisions in everyday life concerning health care, disease prevention and health promotion to maintain or improve quality of life during the life course.
>
> (WHO, 2013, p4)

Our understanding of measuring health literacy has evolved from measuring one aspect of health literacy, for example, literacy and numeracy (Dumenci et al., 2014; Rowlands et al., 2015), towards measuring it in a multi-dimensional way (Sørensen et al., 2012; McCormack et al., 2017; Degan et al., 2019). There is no 'gold standard' approach in capturing the complexity of health literacy as a construct. For example, Degan et al. (2019) have used the Health Literacy Questionnaire (Osbourne et al., 2013). Below is the Sørensen et al. (2012) description of four competencies that are crucial dimensions in the process related to health literacy: accessing, understanding, appraising and applying information (Table 5.1).

DOI: 10.4324/9781003187882-7

Table 5.1 Competencies in the process of health literacy

1   *Access* refers to the ability to seek, find and obtain health information.
2   *Understand* refers to the ability to comprehend the health information that is accessed.
3   *Appraise* describes the ability to interpret, filter, judge and evaluate the health information that has been accessed.
4   *Apply* refers to the ability to communicate and use the information to make a decision to maintain and improve health.

Sørensen et al. (2012, p. 9).

This was developed from a systematic review and integration of definitions and models and includes examining these competencies within the context of health care, disease prevention and health promotion.

This chapter will examine interventions to improve health literacy within a social ecological model developed by McCormack et al. (2017). This social ecological approach involves five multilevel intervention strategies for addressing low health literacy and promoting patient engagement (see Table 5.2). Batterham et al. (2016), who examine levels at which health literacy can be measured, also use this multilevel approach. Within health settings this included individual patients, patient groups and individual health services; and within community and population settings this included local areas, national surveys to compare regions and groups and countries for international comparisons.

Significance of health literacy

Health literacy remains a significant problem within Europe and North America for people with limited health literacy since they have lower rates of health service use and worse health outcomes than people with higher health literacy (Berkman et al., 2011; Bo et al., 2014). In terms of prevalence, almost 48% of the European population has limited health literacy (Sorensen et al., 2015) with a prevalence ranging from 36% in the Netherlands to 62% in Bulgaria. Low health literacy can clearly be linked to health disparities, with greater association with sociodemographic variables such as ethnic minorities, lower educational attainment and older age (Paasche-Orlow et al., 2005; Berkman et al., 2011). Therefore, poor health outcomes originating from limited health literacy can reflect a fundamental injustice of a healthcare system (Volandes & Paasche-Orlow, 2007). As Berkman et al. (2011, p97) comment:

> Low health literacy was consistently associated with more hospitalizations; greater use of emergency care; lower receipt of mammography screening and influenza vaccine; poorer ability to demonstrate taking medications appropriately; poorer ability to interpret labels and health messages; and, among elderly persons, poorer overall health status and higher mortality rates. Poor health literacy partially explains racial disparities in some outcomes.

Patients with higher levels of health literacy also have rates of adherence to medical advice that are, on average, 14% higher than patients who have low health

Table 5.2 Factors that influence and interventions that may improve health literacy and patient engagement (in relation to end of life and substance use), by level of the social ecological model (adapted from McCormack et al., 2017)

Level of influence and influential factors	*Interventions to address limitations*
Individual level Health-related knowledge; attitudes, health beliefs including fatalism, perceptions of risk and benefit; values and preferences for level of involvement; health literacy skills	1 For issues like fatalism, seek psychological support since mental health problems may be underlying reasons for disengagement for people using substances. 2 Address misconceptions about pain management. 3 Use of plain language, best practices and clear communication principles in written communications that specifically address the needs of people who use substances. 4 Data visualisation strategies, realistic health education, adapted to individual need. 5 Delivering care in settings familiar to individuals (e.g. hostel-based care, home care, where possible). Patient decision aids.
Interpersonal level Communication skills, social support	1 Patient-centred communication, active listening, teach-back, awareness of the context of social support. 2 Pre-plan care and consider how to manage complexity in order to enable provision of the best possible care and ensure that any staff anxieties are acknowledged and discussed. 3 Patient and family/friend support groups: assess what family support is available there for people in their own right. Community health workers, shared decision-making.
Organisational level Infrastructure planning and implementation, system integration and coordination	1 Staff training in palliative care for drug and alcohol services, and in drug and alcohol awareness for palliative care services. 2 Coordinated interdisciplinary team-based care with a key worker, physical environment layout and signage, workforce initiatives (e.g. health coaches, navigators). 3 Sharing of electronic medical records. 4 Involving people with lived experience to participate meaningfully in designing, assessing and evaluating services is important. 5 Developing organisational level policies that reflect an awareness of the overlap between substance use and palliative/end of life care. One example would be substance use services including a regular self-audit of people attending the service using a tool such as Supportive Palliative Care Indicator Tool (SPICT) (https://www.spict.org.uk/).

(Continued)

Level of influence and influential factors	*Interventions to address limitations*
Community level Community-based programmes, integration of public health and health care systems	1 Public awareness to address stigma related to substance use, death awareness. Social campaigns (e.g. Dying Matters), e-health communication (e.g. apps and websites with health information in plain language relevant to people using substances) and community-based participatory research. 2 Assertive outreach and engagement with, for example, people who have dropped out of care or people needing home visits. 3 Considering appropriate health care environments may help to combat loneliness and enhance belonging for people with substance use problems with life-limiting conditions.
Macro level Public policy, regulation, legal regulations and incentives, accountability, reliance on evidence-based policies	1 End of Life Care Strategy (2008), NICE (2011), Leadership Alliance for the Care of Dying People (2014), to encourage early referral and recognition of end-of-life conditions, as well as value-based care. 2 A move away from a 'recovery'-based approach to one of harm reduction for end-of-life care for people using substances. Adaption and adoption of clinical guidelines that can meet this population's needs.

literacy skills (Miller 2016). Health literacy has a clear impact within a palliative care context, with Nouri et al. (2019) suggesting that this matters more than experience for advance care planning (ACP) knowledge among older adults. Not least because the written material published for advanced care planning requires a high health literacy level in order to navigate and comprehend it. The impact of health literacy can be seen to extend to decision-making at the end of life, with Bélanger et al. (2011) suggesting that low health literacy impedes joint decision-making. Volandes et al. (2008) indicate it is health literacy, not race, that predicts end-of-life care preferences for African Americans, with most palliative care education articles readily available on Google written above national health literacy level recommendations (Prabhu et al., 2017). There is therefore a clear need to revise these resources to allow patients and their families to derive the most benefit from such materials.

Health literacy and substance use

People living with problematic substance use often present with numerous co-existing conditions, such as mental health problems, chronic obstructive pulmonary disease and cancer (Witham et al., 2019). There are also higher rates of alcohol-related problems and early death associated with chronic and acute alcohol problems (Taylor et al., 2010; Shield et al., 2014). This has a significant impact in reduced quality of life and is often exacerbated by disengagement from primary healthcare and non-adherence to health recommendations (Witham et al., 2019). Individuals using substances with lower health literacy profiles have poor reading ability which can affect their ability to understand health advice (Andrus and Roth, 2002; Zhang et al., 2014). Yet Degan et al. (2019) found that people using substances with low/moderate literacy were more likely to rate themselves as having 'okay' or 'good' reading ability compared to highly health literate individuals. Degan et al. (2019) also describe how quality of life was significantly higher among people with a higher health literacy profile than individuals with low or moderate health literacy, particularly in relation to psychological distress and self-reported mental health. Family communication and maintaining social networks seems to be related to improved health literacy (Zambrana et al., 2015; Degan et al., 2019). People who lived with family before any treatment for substance use were more likely to have moderate or high health literacy compared to those living alone (Degan et al., 2019).

Health literacy in the context of individuals with substance use problems at the end of life

Limited health literacy is often exacerbated by health and social care professionals' attitudes and stigma (Giandinoto et al., 2018). Within the wider social context, we know that stigma and discrimination are common experiences for people using substances within the UK (Radcliffe and Stevens, 2008; Livingston et al., 2011). This can lead to individuals with problematic substance use being reluctant to access formalised healthcare or concealing their actual substance using behaviour in fear of anticipated discrimination. Because of the perceived judgements associated with substance use, people may also conceal health literacy problems. Within this substance using population, where people are potentially exposed to more discrimination, ascertaining health knowledge and understanding can become particularly problematic.

The case studies highlighted within the following sections of this chapter were generated from data derived from a multiple stranded National Lottery funded project (Galvani et al., 2016). People using substances at the end of life often present late to formalised health and social care services (Stajduhar et al., 2019). This can mean that the acute nature of late presentation often relegates questions of health literacy to an optional exploration if care staff have time. An example of this comes from Rob, aged 42, who had been an injecting drug user since the age of 20. He had periods of abstinence, but never felt able to 'fully' give drugs up. He developed end stage heart failure after endocarditis following intravenous drug use and had emergency open-heart surgery. He comments on the period immediately before hospitalisation:

> It pretty much all started about May this year, I was ill for about ten days with flu-like symptoms but I'm not a man-flu type person and this was quite severe.

> What had struck me, there was other things like vomiting that made me think it wasn't just flu. Just over a week and I went to a friend's and said, 'Do you mind if I stay for a few days? I'm really not feeling good.' I live on my own and I should put that in. I said: 'I'd just feel a bit better if there was somebody to keep an eye on me.' And he said 'Yes', obviously, "Stay as long as you like."
>
> (Ashby et al., 2018, p32)

Rob did not access a doctor or go to the hospital and this typifies the experiences of people using substances. Instead, his first call for support was from a friend. The chronic nature of substance use and the often complex and challenging nature of domestic life for people who are substance dependent, means it may be difficult to explore health literacy with them, particularly when they have limited choices, options and resources. Therefore, an individualised approach to health literacy, whereby the health and social care professional examines knowledge gaps and operationalises solutions in terms of motivation to change may pathologise problem drug use. Such an approach often does not acknowledge the wider contextual nature of heath literacy. For example, Barbara, aged 55, developed a drinking problem as a result of suffering domestic abuse in her former marriage over ten years previously. This realisation of dependency was a process of recognising how it had originated – as Barbara comments: *because of my marriage, drink was my only way that I thought I could cope with the problems that I was going through, which led me to become a full blown alcoholic.* When she was seen by a consultant, a scan indicated end stage liver disease. This came as a shock since she felt well and was not given any advice to the contrary by health professionals prior to this consultation. This is not to argue poor communication is not a common feature of end-of-life care generally (Broom et al., 2014), but rather that this population is particularly vulnerable to miscommunication. Health literacy within this context is challenging due to mistrust and the potential for stigma and social discrimination as Barbara comments:

> [Gastroenterologist] he's treated me as another person who just drank. He didn't know my background, he didn't know I was abused mentally and physically by my husband ... I was beaten, he didn't know that. He just saw a six stone alcoholic and that is all he could see because he had no delving into my past.
>
> (Ashby et al., 2018, p51)

Health professionals and people using substances, partly due to not recognising dying and a fear of a negative response in raising the topic, often avoid effective conversations about death awareness (Ebenau et al., 2020), an important aspect of health literacy at the end of life. This is often exacerbated by closed communication by people using substances when talking about end-of-life care planning (Ebenau et al., 2019). This population are particularly vulnerable to avoidance behaviours related to fear of stigma from health and social care professionals (Livingston et al., 2011). They also often experience fractured familial social ties caused by their long-term substance use that can further isolate them and offer little opportunity to explore end-of-life care (Ebenau et al., 2020). The times when opportunities are present to explore more frank 'long-term' conversations are often squandered. For example, Daniel has been a heroin user since the age of 15 and has end stage alcoholic liver disease. He comments on poor communication with health professionals within acute care:

> No, I don't ask the questions, but they weren't forthcoming. I mean they could have said, 'You're going to die in the next ten years because of what you've done. Oh, and by the way if you carry on drinking, you'll not get the next five years.' They could have said that.
>
> (Ashby et al., 2018, p41)

In summary, problems of health literacy may not be addressed because of stigmatisation by health and social care professionals and this is often characterised by poor communication between both professionals and people using substances. This can be exacerbated by anticipatory discrimination leading to the person using substances to withdraw from perceived judgemental authority figures and remain cautious to self-disclosure. The person using substances may also have memory or capacity problems due to cognitive impairment that means assessing health literacy is complex and time consuming, requiring a comprehensive assessment (Wadd et al., 2013). Finally, this population are more likely to have limited family or carers in supportive networks to help mediate and interpret health information (Wright et al., 2018). This is often within a medical context of late presentation where advance care planning and symptom management may be more challenging to manage for health and social care professionals.

Health literacy in the context of family, friends and formal carers/support workers of people using substances at the end of life

Families' health literacy in navigating complex service provision is often limited, with multiple agency interventions making it challenging to know whom to seek support from (Wright et al., 2018). For example, Peter was living with multiple health conditions including liver failure, cognitive difficulties and problems with his balance (resulting in frequent falls). He had a long history of problematic alcohol use. There were, at one point, ten different health care services involved in his care including a liver medical consultant, liver specialist nurse, chest clinic, physiotherapy, Alcoholics Anonymous, carers, specialist in gastroenterology, drug and alcohol services, GP, social worker and an occupational therapist. Peter received appointment letters, but his family found it challenging to work out whom they were from and what they were about. There was also an assumption that the person with complex problems can: (a) attend multiple appointments, (b) arrange transport to attend or be physically able to attend at that time point, and (c) take family or informal carers who may need to work on appointment days. There appears to be both a lack of effective information, communication and joined up care by health and social care professionals. Families with limited health literacy are often attempting to prioritise the most important appointments (without knowing what the most pressing priorities should be for their family member), as well as simultaneously providing daily care and support while monitoring and reviewing fluctuations in health and social care needs (Stajduhar et al., 2020). Families are expected to invest time and energy working on health literacy, including coordinating appointments that will support and potentially adapt care to meet the needs of their relative's health decline. Navigating this system requires information from formalised services and an awareness of the impact of multi-agency interventions upon both the patient and their social networks (Stajduhar et al., 2019).

Supporting family/informal carers' health literacy also requires health and social care practitioners to be honest about the life-shortening possibility of their relative/friends substance use behaviour (Wright et al., 2018). Without effective communication about harm reduction, relatives may ignore the links between health problems and substance use. One daughter described her father's denial of his detrimental use of alcohol and his insistence that his worsening symptoms were related to his long-term conditions rather than alcohol use. Her father subsequently died in hospital:

> Nothing that was an illness to him was ever connected to his drinking -so it was never couched in those terms.... So that was when he hit his early 50s and then for the next ten years or so, other things started to emerge like Stage 3 kidney failure and then much later, in his sort of early to mid-60s, he developed diabetes mellitus and throughout all of this, he continued to drink.
>
> (Yarwood et al., 2018, p21)

The complexity of health literacy problems for relatives of the individual using substances needs to be acknowledged since there is often underlying emotional distress or mental health problems that can affect a relatives' ability to either seek health or social care or engage with the treatment regimens (Yarwood et al., 2018). Relatives may also have limited impact in affecting behaviour change for the individual using substances because of the long- term health changes that have occurred (Ebenau et al., 2020). For example, heavy alcohol use could have impaired the ability of the person using substances to reflect on making lifestyle changes and so compromise their ability to engage with health interventions. Families may also struggle when conveying health information because of their relatives' denial of the detrimental impact of substances to their health. If health and social care professionals attempt to proactively introduce issues of end-of-life care, then this can facilitate a more constructive conversation between family and the relative (Yarwood et al., 2018). This may include confronting both the denial of the impact of using substances and denial of an end-of-life prognosis.

Health literacy was also an important issue between health and social care practitioners: with staff in drug and alcohol services lacking expertise in end-of-life care, leading to uncertainty and reticence in approaching the subject with people engaging with services who are approaching end of life; while practitioners within hospice or palliative care settings felt ill equipped to manage and support the problems that substance use can often generate (Galvani et al., 2018). This requires effective multidisciplinary training and joint working in order to provide an effective service to those individuals using substances at the end of life. This, for example, could take the form of developing practice guidance on pain and symptom management for people with current or previous use of substances at end of life. Other examples, can take the form of 'death awareness' for those in drug and alcohol services since recognising dying can be challenging for those individuals with potentially multiple chronic conditions. For palliative care services, support could be needed to encourage 'positive prescribing' since there is often an under prescribing of effective pain medication for people using substances at the end of life, often related to the fear of overdosing (Witham et al., 2020).

Strategies to support health literacy

After examining health literacy within the context of both people using substances at the end of life and formal/informal carers of people using substances, we now examine what interventions may support health literacy within this population. Micro strategies to improve health literacy can be helpful. For example, Noordman et al. (2019) found some evidence related to face-to-face strategies involving micro-communication skills, jargon-free written and online materials with a more 'ask and tell' method. However, it may be more effective to examine the issue more ecologically. For example, in Table 5.2 we have interventions based on the social ecological model (McCormack et al., 2017). This locates the individual within a social and policy context and acknowledges that health inequalities require more than just interventions at an individual level to address problems of health literacy. Interventions at different levels provide what McCormack et al. (2017) describes as an 'accumulation strategy'. The impact of these interventions at different levels accumulates to effect a common pathway that has significance in potentially improving health literacy and increasing engagement. These accumulative approaches are then subsequently moderated or amplified by another intervention and can facilitate the 'boosting' of the message to enact effective change. Finally, a 'cascade' strategy enables an intervention at one level to influence an outcome through one or more levels and this allows a convergence of the different interventions, 'reinforcing each other and changing interaction patterns' (McCormack et al., 2017, p11).

Paasche-Orlow & Wolf (2010) also examine health literacy within a wider social framework, acknowledging the influence that health disparities have when attempting to address low health literacy. They assert the importance of measuring health literacy by integrating its assessment through improving patient education while exploring how to simplify complex health care systems. This is particularly important since as Volandes & Paasche-Orlow (2007, p5) comment:

> Despite decades of reports exhibiting that the healthcare system is overly complex, unneeded complexity remains commonplace and endangers the lives of patients, especially those with limited health literacy.

Addressing the problems of both access to and utilisation of formalised health care systems is integral to improving health literacy and requires both interdisciplinary and patient/carer collaboration through education and training. We can explore and unpack this complexity further by using a practice example of health literacy and pain management within palliative and end-of-life care for people using substances. We can take a social ecological approach to this topic to explore how health literacy can influence pain management (see Figure 5.1).

Limited health literacy in relation to pain management remains a complex challenge. There may be a requirement for training and workforce development. For health and social care professionals, support and training may be required on substance use for those working in palliative care, and conversely, palliative care training may be needed by practitioners working in drug and alcohol services. This training and support can extend to non-traditional contexts at the end of life. For example, people using substances may experience homelessness and have important social networks within a shelter. In this context, a shelter support worker may give primary support and will need information about pain management if the person is at the end of life and prefers to stay in the shelter (Witham et al., 2019). For the person using substances at end of life, they may be concerned that their pain will not be managed due to discrimination or stigma. They may also be reluctant to take opioids if in recovery, since it can be associated with the negative impact substances had within their lives when using (Witham et al., 2019). This requires support and information to address these concerns.

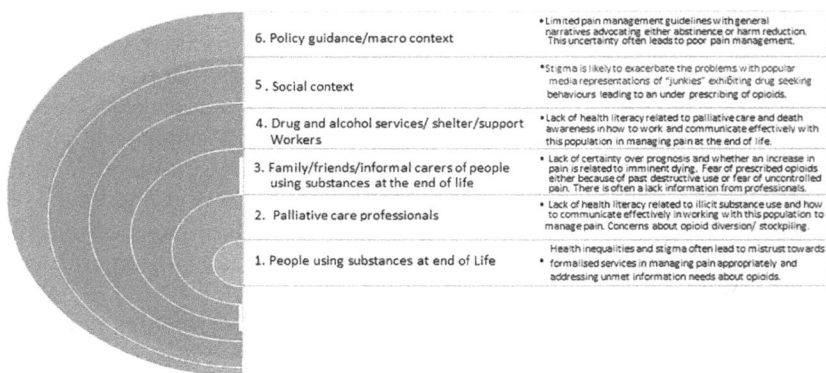

6. Policy guidance/macro context	• Limited pain management guidelines with general narratives advocating either abstinence or harm reduction. This uncertainty often leads to poor pain management.
5. Social context	• Stigma is likely to exacerbate the problems with popular media representations of "junkies" exhibiting drug seeking behaviours leading to an under prescribing of opioids.
4. Drug and alcohol services/ shelter/support Workers	• Lack of health literacy related to palliative care and death awareness in how to work and communicate effectively with this population in managing pain at the end of life.
3. Family/friends/informal carers of people using substances at the end of life	• Lack of certainty over prognosis and whether an increase in pain is related to imminent dying. Fear of prescribed opioids either because of past destructive use or fear of uncontrolled pain. There is often a lack information from professionals.
2. Palliative care professionals	• Lack of health literacy related to illicit substance use and how to communicate effectively in working with this population to manage pain. Concerns about opioid diversion/ stockpiling.
1. People using substances at end of Life	• Health inequalities and stigma often lead to mistrust towards formalised services in managing pain appropriately and addressing unmet information needs about opioids.

Figure 5.1 Conceptual circle of the complexity of health literacy related to pain management at the end of life for people who use substances.

Family and peers may have specific health literacy needs that should be addressed in relation to pain management. This is important since there may be limited opportunities to access effective social care, exacerbating existing health inequalities for these populations. This may also be more challenging if there are negative perceptions that family or peers could potentially steal or divert medicines (Galvani et al., 2018). Health literacy at a community/public health level may be required to prevent labelling the behaviour of this population at the end of life as 'drug-seeking', rather than expressing a legitimate need to address painful symptoms. There is limited availability of policy guidance for opioid titration for people using substances at the end of life (there is some local guidance, e.g. Finnegan et al., 2009). This means that this population are often under prescribed effective pain relief (Barclay et al., 2014; Carmichael et al., 2016).

Conclusion

Health literacy is of key importance in health outcomes and people using substances at the end of life can experience multiple health inequalities. This creates a complex challenge to address health literacy needs since it requires navigating both the needs of the individual, the needs of their social network and the interdisciplinary needs of formalised services involved in the person's care. The wider cultural context of stigma and discrimination often experienced by people using substances means addressing limited health literacy depends on relationship building by health and social care professionals and exhibiting effective non-judgemental communication skills. It is also a wider issue than just addressing individual health information needs, since the intersectionality of substance use with areas such as mental health and social deprivation requires attention to overlapping factors such as organisational issues of access and discrimination, class, gender, race and the interplay with health inequalities. This requires health and social care professionals to address problems of health literacy related to both themselves and people using substances in terms of accessing health information and supporting the understanding of that information (including its appraisal and application) in ways that meaningfully reflect the potential complexity of people using substances at the end of life.

References

Andrus, M.R. and Roth, M.T. (2002) 'Health literacy: A review.' *Pharmacotherapy*, 22(3), pp. 282–302. DOI: 10.1592/phco.22.5.282.33191.

Ashby, J., Wright, S. and Galvani, S. (2018) *Interviews with people at the end of life: End of life care for people with alcohol and drug problems.* Manchester, Manchester Metropolitan University. https://endoflifecaresubstanceuse.com/wp-content/uploads/2018/11/end-of-life-care-for-people-with-substance-use-pwe-full-report-final.pdf [Accessed 21st March 2022].

Australian Bureau of Statistics. (2006) *Health literacy* (Cat. No. 4233.0) Canberra, Australian Bureau of Statistics. Accessed: https://www.ausstats.abs.gov.au/ausstats/subscriber.nsf/0/73ED158C6B14BB5ECA2574720011AB83/$File/42330_2006.pdf [Accessed 3rd July 2020].

Barclay, J.S., Owens, J.E. and Blackhall, L.J. (2014) 'Screening for substance abuse risk in cancer patients using the opioid risk tool and urine drug screen.' *Supportive Care in Cancer*, 22(7), pp. 1883–1888. DOI: 10.1007/s00520-014-2167-6

Batterham, R.W., Hawkins, M., Collins, P.A., Buchbinder, R. and Osborne R.H. (2016) 'Health literacy: Applying current concepts to improve health services and reduce health inequalities.' *Public Health*, 132, pp. 3–12. DOI: 10.1016/j.puhe.2016.01.001

Bélanger, E., Rodriguez, C. and Groleau, D. (2011) 'Shared decision-making in palliative care: A systematic mixed studies review using narrative synthesis.' *Palliative Medicine*, 25, pp. 242–261. DOI: 10.1177/0269216310389348

Berkman, N.D., Davis, T.C. and McCormack, L. (2010) 'Health literacy: What is it?' *Journal of Health Communication*, 15, pp. 9–19. DOI: 10.1080/10810730.2010.499985

Berkman, N.D., Sheridan, S.L., Donahue, K.E., Halpern, D.J. and Crotty, K. (2011) 'Low literacy and health outcomes: An updated systematic review.' *Annuals of Internal Medicine*, 155, pp. 97–107. DOI: 10.7326/0003-4819-155-2-201107190-00005

Bo, A., Friis, K., Osborne, R.H and Maindal, H.T. (2014) 'National indicators of health literacy: Ability to understand health information and to engage actively with healthcare providers - A population-based survey among Danish adults.' *BMC Public Health*, 14, p. 1095. DOI: 10.1186/1471-2458-14-1095

Broom, A., Kirby, E., Good, P., Wootton, J. and Adams, J. (2014) 'The troubles of telling: Managing communication about the end of life.' *Qualitative Health Research*, 24, pp. 151–162. DOI: 10.1177/1049732313519709

Carmichael, A.N., Morgan, L. and DelFabbro, E. (2016) 'Identifying and assessing the risk of opioid abuse in patients with cancer: An integrative review.' *Substance Abuse Rehabilitation*, 7, pp. 71–79. DOI: 10.2147/SAR.S85409

Degan, T.J., Kelly, P.J., Robinson, L.D. and Deane, F.P. (2019) 'Health literacy in substance use disorder treatment: A latent profile analysis.' *Journal of Substance Abuse Treatment*, 96, pp. 46–52. DOI: 10.1016/j.jsat.2018.10.009

Dumenci, L., Matsuyama, R., Riddle, D, L., Cartwright, L., A., Perera, R., A., Chung, H. and Siminoff, L.A. (2014) 'Measurement of cancer health literacy and identification of patients with limited cancer health literacy.' *Journal of Health Communication*, 19(sup2), pp. 205–224. DOI: 10.1080/10810730.2014.943377

Ebenau, A., Dijkstra, B., ter Huurne, C. Hasselaar, J., Vissers, K. and Groot, M. (2019) 'Palliative care for people with substance use disorder and multiple problems: A qualitative study on experiences of patients and proxies.' *BMC Palliative Care*, 18, p. 56. DOI: 10.1186/s12904-019-0443-4

Ebenau, A., Dijkstra, B., ter Huurne, C., Hasselaar, J., Vissers, K. and Groot, M. (2020) 'Palliative care for patients with substance use disorder and multiple problems: A qualitative study on experiences of healthcare professionals, volunteers and experts-by-experience.' *BMC Palliative Care*, 19, p. 8. DOI: 10.1186/s12904-019-0502-x

Finnegan, C., Chapman, L., Fountain, A. and Cannell, L. (2009) *Guidelines for the management of palliative care patients with a history of substance misuse.* https://drive.google.com/file/d/1_imnxnUjU2mcE9pqXqLir0oYeD-6dexI/view [Accessed 19th August 2020].

Galvani, S., Dance, C. and Wright, S. (2018) *Experiences of hospice and substance use professionals: End of life care for people with alcohol and drug problems.* Manchester, Manchester Metropolitan University. https://endoflifecaresubstanceuse.com/wp-content/uploads/2018/11/end-of-life-care-for-people-with-substance-use-professionals-perspective-full-report.pdf [Accessed 21st March 2022].

Galvani, S., Tetley, J., Haigh, C., Webb, L., Yarwood, G., Ashby, J., Duncan, F. and Witham, G. (2016) End of life care for people with alcohol and other drug problems: An exploratory study. *BMJ Supportive & Palliative Care.* DOI: 10.1136/bmjspcare-2016-001204.23

Giandinoto, J-A., Stephenson, J. and Edward, K-L. (2018) 'General hospital health professionals' attitudes and perceived dangerousness towards patients with comorbid mental and physical health conditions: Systematic review and meta-analysis.' *Mental Health Nursing*, pp. 942–955. DOI: 10.1111/inm.12433

Livingston, J.D., Milne, T., Fang, M.L. and Amari, E. (2011) 'The effectiveness of interventions for reducing stigma related to substance use disorders: A systematic review.' *Addiction*; 107, pp. 39–50. DOI: 10.1111/j.1360-0443.2011.03601.x

McCormack, L., Thomas, V., Lewis, M.A. and Rudd, R. (2017) 'Improving low health literacy and patient engagement: A social ecological approach.' *Patient Education and Counseling*, 100, pp. 8–13. DOI: 10.1016/j.pec.2016.07.007

Miller, T.A. (2016) 'Health literacy and adherence to medical treatment in chronic and acute illness: A meta-analysis.' *Patient Education and Counseling*, 99(7), pp. 1079–1086. DOI: 10.1016/j.pec.2016.01.020

Noordman, J., van Vliet L., Kaunang M, van den Muijsenbergh, M., Boland, G. and van Dulmen, S. (2019) 'Towards appropriate information provision for and decision-making with patients with limited health literacy in hospital-based palliative care in Western countries: A scoping review into available communication strategies and tools for healthcare providers.' *BMC Palliative Care*, 18, p. 37. DOI: 10.1186/s12904-019-0421-x

Nouri, S.S., Barnes, D.E., Volow, A.M., McMahan, R.D., Kushel, M., Jin, C., Boscardin, J. and Sudore, R.L. (2019) 'Health literacy matters more than experience for advance care planning knowledge among older adults.' *Journal of American Geriatric Society*, 67, pp. 2151–2156. DOI: 10.1111/jgs.16129

Osborne, R.H., Batterham, R., Elsworth, G.R., Hawkins, M. and Buchbinder, R. (2013) 'The grounded theory, psychometric development and initial validation of the Health Literacy Questionnaire (HLQ).' *BMC Public Health*, 13, p. 658. DOI: 10.1186/1471-2458-13-658

Paasche-Orlow MK, Parker RM, Gazmararian JA, Nielsen-Bohlman LT, Rudd RR. (2005) The prevalence of limited health literacy. *Journal of General Internal Medicine*. (2):175-84. doi: 10.1111/j.1525-1497.2005.40245.x.

Paasche-Orlow, M.K. and Wolf, M.S. (2010) 'Promoting health literacy research to reduce health disparities.' *Journal of Health Communication*, 15:S2, pp. 34–41. DOI: 10.1080/10810730.2010.499994

Prabhu, A.V., Crihalmeanu, T., Hansberry, D.R., Agarwal, N., Glaser, C., Clump, D.A., Heron, D.W. and Beriwal, S. (2017) 'Online Palliative Care and oncology patient education resources through Google: Do they meet national health literacy recommendations?' *Practical Radiation Oncology*, 7(5), pp. 306–310. DOI: 10.1016/j.prro.2017.01.013

Radcliffe, P. and Stevens, A. (2008) 'Are drug treatment services only for 'thieving, junkie scrum bags?' Drug users and the management of stigmatised Identities.' *Social Science Medicine*, 67, pp. 1065–1073. DOI: 10.1016/j.socscimed.2008.06.004

Rowlands, G., Protheroe, J., Winkley, J., Richardson, M., Seed, T.P. and Rudd, R. (2015) 'A mismatch between population health literacy and the complexity of health information: An observational study.' *British Journal of General Practice*, 65(635), pp. 379–386. DOI: 10.3399/bjgp15X685285.

Shield, K.D., Parry, C. and Rehm, J. (2014) 'Chronic diseases and conditions related to alcohol use.' *Alcohol Research*, 35(20), pp. 155–171. DOI: 2014–07285-006

Sorensen, K., Peilkan, J.M., Rothlin, F., Ganahl, K., Sionska, Z., Doyle, G., Fullam, J., Kondilis, B., Agrafiotis, D., Uiters, E., Falcon, M., Mensing, M., Tchamov, K., van den Broucke, S. and Brand, H. (2015) On behalf of the HLS-EU consortium. 'Health literacy in Europe: Comparative results of the European health literacy survey (HLS-EU).' *European Journal of Public Health*, 25, pp. 1053–1058. DOI: 10.1093/eurpub/ckv043

Sørensen, K., Van den Broucke, S., Fullam, J., Slonska, Z., Brand, H. and (HLS-EU) Consortium Health Literacy Project European. (2012) 'Health literacy and public health: A systematic review and integration of definitions and models.' *BMC Public Health*, 12, p. 80. DOI: 10.1186/1471-2458-12-80

Stajduhar, K I., Giesbrecht, M., Mollison, A., Dosani, N. and McNeil, R. (2020) 'Caregiving at the margins: An ethnographic exploration of family caregivers experiences providing care for structurally vulnerable populations at the end-of-life.' *Palliative Medicine*, 34(7), pp. 946–953. DOI: 10.1177/0269216320917875

Stajduhar, K.I., Mollison, A., Giesbrecht, M. McNeil, R., Pauly, B., Reimer-Kirkham, S., Showler, G., Meagher, C., Kvakic, K., Gleave, D., Teal, T., Rose, C., Showler, C. and Rounds, K. (2019) '"Just too busy living in the moment and surviving": Barriers to accessing health care for structurally vulnerable populations at end-of-life.' *BMC Palliative Care*, 18, p. 11. DOI: 10.1186/s12904-019-0396-7

Taylor, B., Irving, H.M., Kanteres, F., Room, R., Borgen, G., Cherpitel, C. and Rehm, J. (2010) 'The more you drink, the harder you fall: A systematic review and meta-analysis of how acute alcohol consumption and injury or collision risk increase together.' *Drug & Alcohol Dependence*, 110(1–2), pp. 108–116. DOI: 10.1016/j.drugalcdep.2010.02.011

Volandes, A.E. and Paasche-Orlow, M.K. (2007) 'Health literacy, health inequality and a just healthcare system.' *The American Journal of Bioethics*, 7(11), pp. 5–10. DOI: 10.1080/15265160701638520

Volandes, A.E., Paasche-Orlow, M.K., Gillick, M.R., Cook, E.F., Shaykevich, S., Abbo, E.D. and Lehmann, L. (2008) 'Health literacy not race predicts end-of-life care preferences.' *Journal of Palliative Medicine*, 11(5), pp. 754–762. DOI: 10.1089/jpm.2007.0224

Wadd, S., Randall, J., Thake, A., Edwards, K., Galvani, S., McCabe, L. and Coleman, A (2013) *Alcohol misuse and cognitive impairment in older people.* https://s3.eu-west-2.amazonaws.com/files.alcoholchange.org.uk/documents/FinalReport_0110.pdf [Accessed 18th August 2020].

WHO Regional Office for Europe. (2013) *Health literacy: The solid facts.* Copenhagen: WHO Regional Office for Europe. https://apps.who.int/iris/bitstream/handle/10665/128703/e96854.pdf [Accessed 8th March 2022].

Witham, G., Peacock, M. and Galvani, S. (2019) 'End of life care for people with alcohol and drug problems: Findings from a rapid evidence assessment.' *Health and Social Care in the Community*, 27(5), e637–e650. DOI: 10.1111/hsc.12807.

Witham, G., Yarwood, G., Wright, S., and Galvani, S. (2020) 'An ethical exploration of the narratives surrounding substance use and pain management at the end of life: A discussion paper.' *Nursing Ethics*, 27(5), pp. 1344–1354. DOI: 10.1177/0969733019871685

Wright, S., Yarwood, G.A., Templeton, L. and Galvani, S. (2018) *Experiences of families, friends, carers: Phase 1 end of life care for people with alcohol and drug problems.* Manchester, Manchester Metropolitan University. https://endoflifecaresubstanceuse.com/wp-content/uploads/2018/11/end-of-life-care-for-people-with-substance-use-family-strand-phase-1-report.pdf [Accessed 21st March 2022].

Yarwood, G.A., Wright, S., Templeton, L. and Galvani, S. (2018) *End of life care for people with alcohol and other drug problems: Qualitative analysis of primary interviews with family members, friends and carers.* Manchester, Manchester Metropolitan University. https://endoflifecaresubstanceuse.com/wp-content/uploads/2018/11/end-of-life-care-for-people-with-substance-use-family-report-phase-2-final-full-report1.pdf [Accessed 21st March 2022].

Zambrana, R., Meghea, C., Talley, C., Hammad, A., Lockett, M. and Williams, K. (2015) 'Association between family communication and health literacy among underserved racial/ethnic women.' *Journal of Health Care for the Poor and Underserved*, 26(2), pp. 391–405. DOI: 10.1353/hpu.2015.0034.

Zhang, N.J., Terry, A. and McHorney, C.A. (2014) 'Impact of health literacy on medication adherence: A systematic review and meta-analysis.' *Annals of Pharmacotherapy*, 48(6), pp. 741–751. DOI: 10.1177/1060028014526562.

6 Learning disabilities and substance use at the end of life

Listening to the unheard

Gary Witham and Sarah Galvani

Introduction

People with learning disabilities are an ageing population. As with the general population, they are also living longer due to social and medical improvements (Emerson et al., 2011). This longevity is associated with an increase in chronic, life-threatening diseases such as cancer, chronic obstructive airway disease or heart failure (Heslop et al., 2014) and increasing social care needs such as housing and social support (NICE, 2018). Consideration must, therefore, be given to how their palliative and end-of-life care needs can be met (Watson et al., 2017; Voss et al., 2020).

Globally, learning disability affects about 1% of the population (Maulik et al., 2011) with mild, moderate, severe and profound learning disabilities affecting about 85%, 10%, 4% and 2% of that 1% population, respectively (King et al., 2009). Learning disabilities can be defined as:

> a significantly reduced ability to understand new or complex information, to learn new skills (impaired intelligence) along with a reduced ability to cope independently (impaired social functioning). The onset of disability is considered to have started before adulthood, with a lasting effect on development.
>
> (Department of Health (DH), 2001)

This definition includes intelligence quotient (IQ) and functional aspects that make it distinct from the term 'learning difficulties' (Department of Health, 2001). It affects experiential, social and academic learning. There is significant variation in the degree of impairment people with learning disabilities experience in both intelligence and social functioning with subsequent independence and social support predicated on this.

The prevalence of substance use by people with learning disabilities is not known. Taggart et al. (2006) estimated it at 0.8% of the population with learning disabilities, but acknowledged the figure was likely to be an under-estimate. While this prevalence is likely to be lower than the general population, the group most likely to use alcohol and drugs are people with mild learning difficulties who are not in touch with formalised services (McLaughlin et al., 2009; DH, 2016)). This group may be more likely to develop dependency due to peer pressure (Chapman and Wu,

DOI: 10.4324/9781003187882-8

2012) and a propensity to sustain and emulate behaviours they find difficult to alter (McGillicuddy, 2006; Dance and Galvani, 2014). They are sometimes also targeted for drug use, either by others who persuade them to buy drugs or by dealers who want to use their premises (often known as 'cuckooing') (McCarthy et al., 2016). They also may have greater access to substances with greater social freedoms compared to people requiring more support and potentially more restricted social environments (Day et al., 2016). Problematic substance use within this population may be exacerbated by isolation, poor coping abilities and limited social skills (Hammink et al., 2015).

This chapter will explore the challenges of supporting someone with a learning disability using substances at the end of life through a case study approach. The case study is based on an interview with Grace, the sister of Peter, a man with a learning disability who used substances. We will examine the wider context of health inequalities and discrimination and specifically the context and recognition of dying for people living with a learning disability using substances. We will explore the communication challenges between the person with learning disabilities, their family and social network and consider how interdisciplinary working by health and social care professionals can influence care delivery. We will further explore choice and decision-making at the end of life and how substance use can impede decision-making for people with learning disabilities.

Box 6.1 Case study: Peter

Peter was 32 when he died of end stage renal failure. He had a learning disability and had further cognitive challenges caused by a road traffic accident ten years prior to his death which had caused brain damage and left him without function in one arm. He also had type 1 diabetes that was poorly controlled and suffered from anxiety and depression. After the accident he started to use substances frequently and had, over the years, self-harmed and attempted suicide. He had been referred to mental health services, but his family felt this had not been effective. There had been limited agency contact with his family and poor health professional communication and assessment for Peter. Peter would frequently miss hospital and social care appointments because he would forget, and his family were not informed of these appointments despite wanting to help him access support. As a result, he had limited formal service provision. He was also a victim of violence and abuse but refused to report it to the police. In the last year of his life his self-management of his diabetes was particularly poor: leading to poor vision, difficulty mobilising and frequent seizures. This led to end stage renal failure. His sister, Grace, felt his poor diabetic management was a form of self-harm, linked to his mental health. Health professionals, however, interpreted his poor diabetic control in the same way as his substance use: as a 'lifestyle choice' – leading to limited agency intervention. Peter was found dead by Grace when she came to visit him in his rented accommodation.

Health inequalities, discrimination and learning disabilities

Life expectancy for people with learning disabilities remains significantly lower than the general population (Emerson et al., 2014), with the UK Learning Disability Review Programme establishing in 2017 that the median age of death was 47 years old for people with severe and profound disabilities and 63 years old for those with mild or moderate learning disabilities. The UK Care Quality Commission (CQC) (2016) reviewed inequalities in end-of-life care for people with learning disabilities and found that they were at risk of poorer care at the end of life as a result of inadequate needs assessment. The CQC also found people with learning disabilities had challenges accessing specialist palliative care services, with limited advance care planning and coordination of care (Heslop et al., 2013; McLaughlin et al., 2014).

People with learning disabilities are open to significantly more discrimination and abuse, including physical violence, than those without a learning disability (Dammeyer and Chapman, 2018). Asamoah et al. (2009) examined general public attitudes within the United Kingdom towards people with learning disabilities and alcohol use by using vignettes. Participants were randomised and presented with separate vignettes related to alcohol (as round one) and learning disability (round two). The research found comparable levels of stigma associated with both learning disabilities and alcoholism as separate conditions. This raises the question as to whether there is increased stigma for people where both substance use and learning disabilities are present. This may synergistically combine into new and more harmful modes of oppression rather than just an accumulation as indicated in the intersectionality of race and gender: the 'double jeopardy' of marginalised communities (Levin et al., 2002). In the case study above, Peter's sister (Grace) reported that he had received facial injuries from a suspected fight although Peter refused to report this to the police. According to Grace, Peter remained isolated in rented accommodation and tended to just interact with people selling illicit drugs.

Discrimination can also come from health professionals. In a systematic review of mainstream health professionals' attitudes to people with learning disabilities, Pelleboer-Gunnink et al. (2017) found stigmatisation was common, arising from a lack of knowledge and familiarity with this population. People with learning disabilities were seen as different, strange, intimidating, funny or childlike. Only limited adjustments were made to daily care routines to cater for their individual support needs. There was also an increase in stress and anxiety and a lack of confidence by health professionals in supporting people with a learning disability in comparison to those without a learning disability. According to Grace, Peter's interactions with health and social care professionals highlighted an inflexibility in their offer of care and a failure to adapt to the cognitive challenges he faced. Health and social care professionals also failed to recognise the consequences for him of not involving his family more centrally in his care. As Grace comments:

> ...apparently there was a referral to a drug worker which was not passed onto us. He couldn't manage his own affairs: if he had appointments, he'd never

go – either doesn't want to go or wouldn't tell anyone, so we missed that. It's like I say, it was made very clear that he couldn't function on his own, so we needed to be informed. But most of the time, we weren't informed and then it was like: 'He's missed another appointment'.

Substance use alone carries clear negative stereotyping (Livingston et al., 2011) with stigmatising attitudes from professionals that can impede access to both primary and acute care (Ashby et al., 2018). There is also clear evidence of inequalities in the provision of healthcare for people with learning disabilities (Cobigo et al., 2013; Emerson and Hatton, 2013). This relates to both general healthcare provision and specialist palliative care, in particular relating to poor access and quality of care, lack of advance care planning and diagnostic overshadowing (where physical ill-health is attributed to the learning disability and therefore not investigated). Subsequently there are delays in accessing hospice care, often exacerbated by inadequate knowledge of people with learning disabilities among hospice staff, poor communication between professionals and between professionals and family members, and issues surrounding informed consent (Friedman et al., 2012). Grace felt her brother faced discrimination in terms of access and commented:

I did say to Social Services quite a lot, "What cost are you putting on my brother's life?" And that's it! "He's not worthy enough for your money." And that's what they were saying to me, and I told them where it would end up. And sure, some people get lucky and get what they want, but it's on an individual basis. They're judging people and they're cherry picking who they want to treat. So, some people's lives are worth more than others and that's not the way it should be.

Identification and assessment of substance use and dying

The challenges of identification and assessment are significant where there is an intersection of learning disabilities, substance use and end-of-life care. For example, Taggart et al. (2006) sent questionnaires to both learning disability and drug and alcohol teams within Northern Ireland. They reported 67 learning disability service users who were known to use substances. However, the need for intervention and support was not established through usual care planning and was often unacknowledged within these two services. There are no validated tools for assessing problematic substance use among people with learning disabilities. Existing tools for assessing substance use are not in a format and level that can be easily understood by someone with learning disabilities. These challenges are reflected in Peter's care since there should have been assessment and identification relating to four overlapping needs including his mental health problems. For Peter, self-harm, suicidal ideation, depression and anxiety both intersected with his substance use and affected his end-of-life care (see Chapter 7 regarding mental health). This ability to assess and identify needs on an interdisciplinary level remains challenging; for Peter, this meant that his care was piecemeal and

fragmented. The ability to adequately assess risk and confidently ask more pertinent questions to facilitate his meaningful engagement did not feature in his care.

Peter's experience was of delay in his diagnosis. His family had reported to his
GP that his health was deteriorating over the previous two years, but no clear
assessment process was identified. As his sister, Grace, comments:

> He went to the doctors. Eventually, we got sent to a kidney specialist and he's got
> Stage 5 kidney disease. And I'm going: 'How can you go from stage nothing to
> stage 5?' And obviously he's showing signs of this already, we've told you! There's
> something not adding up somewhere, but you can't fight the system can you?

There are also difficulties in identifying when someone with learning disabilities
is nearing the end of their lives (Tuffrey-Wijne et al., 2007). Staff working in drug
and alcohol services may also find fluctuating substance use in association with
fluctuating health status more challenging in identifying people in need of end-
of-life care (Galvani et al., 2018). This is important since early discussions and
involvement can potentially facilitate more choice such as treatment options and
preferred place of end-of-life care (Bekkema et al., 2015). Early identification of
palliative care needs was also an important element stemming from a Delphi-based
European consensus exercise that brought together experts in learning disabilities
across Europe. It resulted in a list of 13 norms articulating good practice for people
with learning disabilities (Tuffrey-Wijne et al., 2016). These were: 'equity of access,
communication, recognising the need for palliative care, assessment of total needs,
symptom management, end-of-life decision-making, involving those who matter,
collaboration, support for family/carers, preparing for death, bereavement support,
education/training and developing/managing services'. Vrijmoeth et al. (2018b)
state they have not, however, often been achieved in a timely manner within clinical practice. There have been attempts to develop screening tools with Vrijmoeth
et al. (2018a, 2018b) developing the PALLI tool (PALLIative care: learning to identify in people with intellectual disabilities). This tool is designed to screen people
with learning disabilities for deteriorating health (over a three-to-six-month time
period), with a view to indicating impending end of life (Christians et al., 2016).

Communication challenges

One of the communication challenges that impact on people with learning disability at the end of life relates to the confidence of care staff to have conversations about dying with them. For example, Tuffrey-Wijne and Rose (2017) found
that staff working in learning disability services found open communication about
death and dying very hard and the tendency was to avoid those conversations. This
was often predicated on fear and distress around death based more on personal life
experiences of staff than the needs of the person with learning disabilities. It was
also influenced by the organisational culture – with managers being important role
models in supporting open conversations. In Peter's care, there was a clear lack of
communication about dying and little thought as to how that information would be
conveyed. Grace comments on when the doctor talked to Peter about his prognosis:

I don't think that anyone had explained it properly to him. … He had learning difficulties. He's got a brain injury … I think when you get an end-of-life diagnosis like that – which it is an end-of-life diagnosis – they should come with some form of counselling. Again, that was never offered. You've got told that you've got ten years max. It's very cruel, I think.

There are also reservations about broaching death and dying within specialist alcohol and drug services, with Galvani et al. (2018) finding that staff find it difficult to both recognise dying and have end-of-life conversations. Equally, palliative care staff feel ill-equipped to work with someone with problematic substance use (Galvani et al., 2018), and also with someone with learning disabilities (Cross et al., 2012; Friedman et al., 2012; Read, 2013; Tuffrey-Wijne and McLaughlin, 2015). Staff in a hospice, for example, may find it difficult to differentiate between symptoms associated with the person's health condition and those arising as the consequence of substance use. Indeed, there is some research that indicates individuals with learning disabilities may experience heightened side effects from illicit and prescribed substance use (Degenhardt, 2000), which would make the task of distinguishing between the origins of the presenting symptoms even more difficult to assess. Effective communication between practitioners and people with learning disabilities can be challenging since there is a clear, reported, complexity and multiplicity of need within this group (Tuffrey-Wijne et al., 2016). For example, people using substances with a learning disability, like Peter, are more likely than those who do not use substances to have mood swings, depression and anxiety, more frequent suicidal thoughts and more negative long-term personal relationships (Didden et al., 2009; To et al., 2014). Effective communication is also predicated on building trusting relationships with people with learning disabilities at the end of life. This can be compromised if services are fractured and not working together, or professionals fail to examine the context of a person's life (Ryan et al., 2016).

Effective communication failed to occur for Peter, as Grace comments on the involvement of a specialist nurse:

> They tried to engage but they'd just say: "Peter will not cooperate." But I said to Deborah, his nurse, "But you're not engaging with him. You're dictating to him how he feels and what he does and that's not the way to manage the situation. If you weren't doing that … you would open your eyes and see why, think about why you would be doing this? Why would you not want to have a nice happy life? Why would you not want that?" I was like: "People don't choose that path." I don't think anyone would choose that. It's mental health isn't it? I can't see any drug addict or alcoholic saying "I'm happy." Ever.

Decision-making and informed consent

Problems relating to decision-making and informed consent for people with learning disabilities are also prevalent within the literature (Bernal et al., 2009; Tuffrey-Wijne et al., 2016). These challenges relate to the extent to which someone with learning disabilities has insight into their condition, the treatments offered and possible outcomes. Where substance use is combined with palliative or end-of-life care needs, a lack of insight further compounds the difficulties of communication and consent. For example, Grace describes how Peter's non-engagement with formalised services related to issues of informed consent:

> ... he had one referral and because he didn't turn up to the appointment (because we didn't know about it), it's gone. And you're given one shot at everything. But the whole premise of this was he's got a brain injury and learning difficulties: he cannot manage this – which means he's not competent, so he can't cope on his own...

From the family's perspective, Peter could not give informed consent and, despite him saying he could manage at home, the experience of the family, including his mum, was that he could not. Peter was not involved in his own end-of-life care decisions which made person-centred advance care planning (ACP) difficult to implement. This was because he was neither informed, nor understood the information given to him about the implications of stage 5 renal failure. This lack of appropriate communication is reflected in McKibben et al.'s (2020) study. The health and social care professionals did not have these conversations nor were they providing adequate information in order for people to make informed choices (McKibben et al., 2020). Having early conversations about ACP where substance use is involved is important, since the person's presentation to palliative and end-of-life care may be late. As a result, any care planning at this stage may be within the imminent dying phase, potentially reducing the capacity for informed consent. Therefore, the challenge of working with someone with a learning disability who is dying and may also have memory or cognitive capacity difficulties (that may be exacerbated by substance use) can be a significant hurdle. This requires close working relationships between individuals with learning disabilities, their significant others and interdisciplinary professionals (Ryan et al., 2016). Effective decision-making also requires integrated team working in association with the person with learning disabilities and the building of trust from all parties. This is predicated on open, continuous communication (Voss et al., 2020) and training for interdisciplinary teams to be able to have conversations relevant to informed decision-making, whether this be conversations about substance use (Galvani et al., 2018) or prognostically sensitive information (Cross et al., 2012). Training practitioners and formal carers about 'death awareness' is important to ensure the best possible care for the dying person with learning disabilities, but also to explore professionals' attitudes towards, or reluctance about, initiating end of life or substance use discussions (Galvani et al., 2018; Voss et al., 2020).

Collaborative working

The evidence suggests that better collaboration between services for people with learning disabilities and specialist palliative care services is vital in providing quality care at the end of life (Tuffrey-Wijne et al. 2007; McLaughlin et al. 2009).

The lack of referrals for people with learning disabilities into specialist palliative care suggests limited partnership working (Cross et al., 2012). This is likely to be challenged further with the involvement of another agency, like a drug and alcohol service. Peter was known to social care and to drug and alcohol services. But, apart from a brief prognostic conversation, health professionals did not discuss end-of-life care or Peter's wishes. There appeared to be no communication or collaboration with palliative care services and other agencies.

There is no evidence of routine assessment by professional staff of any overlapping needs for people with substance problems and end-of-life care needs (Galvani et al., 2018). Galvani et al. (2018) found this was often compounded by a lack of confidence or willingness to explore the 'other' need by service providers. This lack of interdisciplinary engagement also relates to people with learning disabilities from both a substance use and end-of-life provider perspective (Friedman et al., 2012; Dance and Galvani, 2014). There is a lack of clear pathways for this population to access the multi-disciplinary services they require to meet their complex needs.

There also appears to be limited collaboration or support given to formal support workers for people with learning disabilities who may lack confidence in their ability to explore an end-of-life prognosis and who wish to protect the person from distress (Bernal et al., 2009). Power and Bartlett (2019) commented on what they call the 'care desert' for older people with learning disabilities within a UK context. They acknowledge that austerity measures in the United Kingdom have meant some previously formalised services have been discontinued, leading to a more precarious level of support for people with learning disabilities which now often comprises only informal support arrangements. Thus, the communication and networking opportunities for carers and people with learning disabilities may be diminished. The opportunity to connect to such networks may be predicated on the effects of age, poverty, gender and disability. Facilitating a connection between formalised services and informal social networks that support people with learning disabilities using substances at the end of life seems crucial to providing effective care and to avoiding late referrals to drug and alcohol services, with people often presenting at crisis point. This requires health and social care staff to recognise the impact of living with, and/or providing care and support for, someone with learning disabilities using substances and for them to examine the impact that the carers have in that person's life. Further, it requires the adoption of proactive and reactive strategies by health and social care staff, including positive behaviour support (PBS) based on harm reduction rather than abstinence (Day et al., 2016).

Public Health England (2016) has produced some evidence-based guidance to promote effective interventions for health and social care staff to support people with learning disabilities who use substances. It advises:

- addiction services and learning disability teams integrate services to provide a link between them
- a personalised approach that tailors interventions to individuals' needs

- interventions and information that meet the particular communication and learning needs of individuals
- people with learning disabilities may benefit from a one-to-one approach rather than group work
- both substance misuse services and learning disability services should screen for misuse problems / learning disabilities at initial assessments
- training for mainstream addiction staff on how to work with people with learning disabilities and how to modify assessment and treatment approaches
- training for learning disabilities professionals around substance misuse
- widening the person's social support networks
- greater family involvement in treatment
- appropriate training and resources for support workers
- access to support services (including bereavement and sexual abuse) that can help people to address the reasons behind their substance misuse
- techniques such as motivational interviewing.

(Public Health England, 2016)

As Public Health England (2016) suggests, improved collaboration extends to the involvement of family members, such as Grace within this case study.

Family involvement

The lack of timely intervention by formalised services caused significant problems. Peter's sister, Grace, describes her attempts to arrange a formal meeting with social services:

> I think they'd re-scheduled it [appointment] for two weeks after he died. But we waited six, seven months for that to happen. In the meantime, he was getting further and further into crisis and every person I spoke to at Social Services, like Mental Health, Social Care were: "That's not our problem, it's someone else's problem." Which is the thing, it's unfortunate.

Family involvement is important within collaborative care for people with learning disabilities at the end of life (Tuffrey-Wijne et al., 2016), although where someone is using substances there could be fractured family relationships (Kepper et al., 2011). Family carers have diverse information needs, with the most frequently expressed needs involving education on the life-limiting condition, palliative care and the illness trajectory (McKibben et al., 2020). In their qualitative study of health and social care professionals and family caregivers from one region of the United Kingdom, McKibben et al. (2020) found that family caregivers were proactive in seeking out information, but that it was often not forthcoming from health and social care professionals. They found that joint working often occurred too late within the relative's illness trajectory to positively impact upon their care. Care staff often acknowledge the importance of active family involvement in their relative's end-of-life care although this does not always translate into practice, leaving families, like Peter's, feeling isolated. The co-existence of substance use with palliative and end-of-life needs is likely to further impede effective collaboration and communication between practitioners, the individual and their family. Discrimination, stigma and fractured relationships between practitioners and the person using substances may leave family carers reluctant to engage with formalised services (Yarwood et al., 2018).

Implications for practice

The key message for practice that is raised by lived experience like Peter's and Grace's, is the urgent need for effective interagency communication that fully acknowledges their expertise. Genuine collaboration requires a key worker to coordinate care and for practitioners at all levels to ensure they have the professionalism to seek out and accept the expertise of significant others like Grace. It is only through proactive and reactive care planning involving all relevant parties that early interventions can potentially support someone with learning disabilities, like Peter, who is using substances at the end of life.

Figure 6.1 highlights a framework for tripartite partnership practice between substance use services, specialist palliative care and learning disability services. This model attempts to overcome some of the barriers to partnership working. This figure includes the context in which palliative care is delivered and examines the connections, learning, action and impacts relating to such tripartite practice. The large arrows point to the core of the model, illustrating optimal palliative care can be provided to people with learning disabilities through partnership.

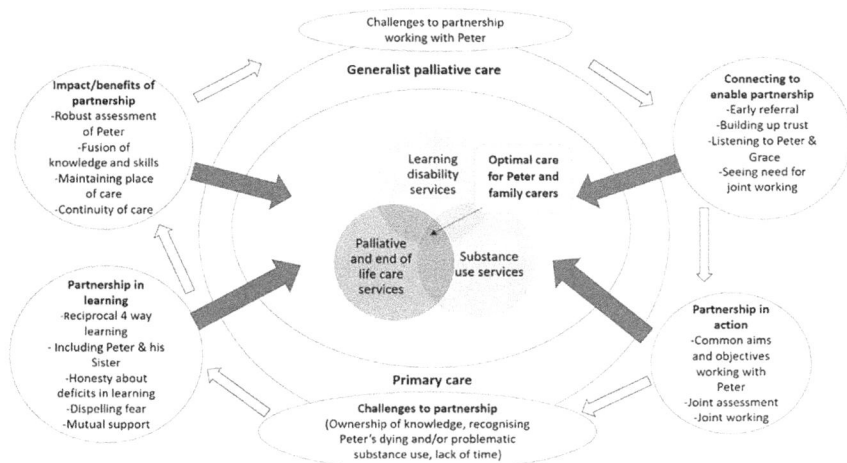

6.1 A framework for partnership practice between substance use services, specialist palliative care and learning disability services (adapted from McLaughlin et al., 2014).

The ovals around the edge are different aspects of good partnership working and some of the challenges to consider in supporting Peter.

In summary, the implications for practice are:

- Interdisciplinary collaboration is a pivotal in providing effective end-of-life care. It may require a key worker to advocate and coordinate a collective, joined up response for someone with learning disabilities using substances at the end of life.
- Liaison with family and significant others needs to occur early in the care journey. They should all be included within multi-disciplinary team meetings and be integral to any interventions from formalised care services to support the person with learning disabilities.
- Information giving should be a process not a single event. It should be in an appropriate format and level for the person with learning disabilities using substances at the end of life. There should be opportunities to ask further questions over a series of meetings.

Conclusion

This chapter has explored end-of-life care for Peter, a man with learning disabilities who also used substances. It has also explored the care given and received by his sister Grace. There are many challenges in supporting Peter and the wider population of people using substances at the end of life. In particular, practitioners need to acknowledge the discrimination and health inequalities that coalesce and give vital insight into the experiences of people with a learning disability. Subsequent problems like mental health and/or substance use can further challenge a coordinated approach by health and social care professionals. This can become particularly acute at the end of life, in both diagnosing dying and assessing the care needs of someone with learning disabilities. In Peter's case, his end of life was not recognised. Developing good practice is critical for providing people with learning disabilities and their families with the opportunity of a good death. Acknowledging and including the family of people with learning disabilities, and other social networks important to the person at end of life, are central to person-centred care. However, it requires a level of interdisciplinary co-ordination that is not often achieved in practice. Engaging any marginalised population requires flexibility of service provision. It also requires professional curiosity to assess and explore the care needs of people who may be initially reluctant to engage with formalised services. This approach can potentially begin to explore, and subsequently meet, the care needs faced by people with learning disabilities using substances at the end of life as well as support their family members who often provide the majority of care.

References

Asamoah, G., Varughese, S. J., Mushtag, S., Butterworth, L., Abraham, A. and Luty, J. (2009) 'A randomised trial of ethnicity and stigmatised attitudes towards learning disability and alcoholism.' *Ethnicity and Inequalities in Health and Social Care*, 2, pp. 11–19. DOI: 10.1108/17570980200900011

Ashby, J., Wright, S. and Galvani, S. (2018) *End of Life Care for People with Alcohol and other Drug Problems: Perspectives of People at their End of Life*. Final Report, Manchester: Manchester Metropolitan University. https://endoflifecaresubstanceuse.com/wp-content/uploads/2018/11/end-of-life-care-for-people-with-substance-use-pwe-full-report-final.pdf [Accessed 21st March 2022].

Bekkema, N., de Veer, A. J., Hertogh, C. M. and Francke, A. L. (2015) 'From activating towards caring': Shifts in care approaches at the end of life of people with intellectual disabilities; a qualitative study of the perspectives of relatives, care-staff and physicians.' *BMC Palliative Care*, 14, p. 33. DOI: 10.1186/s12904-015-0030-2

Care Quality Commission. (2016) *A Different Ending: Addressing Inequalities in End of Life Care—Good Practice Case Studies*. Newcastle upon Tyne: Care Quality Commission. https://www.cqc.org.uk/sites/default/files/20160505%20CQC_EOLC_OVERVIEW_FINAL_3.pdf [Accessed 8th March 2022]

Chapman, S. L. and Wu, L. T. (2012) 'Substance use among individuals with intellectual disabilities.' *Research in Developmental Disabilities*, 33, pp. 1147–1156. DOI: 10.1016/j.ridd.2012.02.009

Christians, M. G., Vrijmoeth, C., Echteld, M., Tonino, M., Festen, D. A., Lantman, H. and Groot, C. M. (2016) *PALLI Study: A Study Protocol for Development and Validation of a Tool for the Identification of People with Intellectual Disabilities Who Are in Need of Palliative Care*. Nijmegen, The Netherlands: Radboudumc. Retrieved from: https://www.researchgate.net/publication/303310869_PALLI_study_a_study_protocol_for_development_and_validation_of_a_tool_for_the_identification_of_people_with_intellectual_disabilities_who_are_in_need_of_palliative_care. 27-02-2021. [Accessed 8th March 2022]

Cobigo, V., Ouellette-Kuntz, H., Balogh, R., Leung, F., Lin, E. and Lunsky, Y. (2013) 'Are cervical and breast cancer screening programmes equitable? The case of women with intellectual and developmental disabilities.' *Journal of Intellectual Disabilities Research*, 57(5), pp. 478–488. DOI: 10.1111/jir.12035

Cross, H., Cameron, M., Marsh, S. and Tuffrey-Wijne, I. (2012) 'Practical approaches toward improving end-of-life care for people with intellectual disabilities: Effectiveness and sustainability.' *Journal of Palliative Medicine*, 15(3), pp. 322–326. DOI: 10.1089/jpm.2011.0132

Dammeyer, J. and Chapman, M. (2018) 'A national survey on violence and discrimination among people with disabilities.' *BMC Public Health*, 18, p. 355. DOI: 10.1186/s12889-018-5277-0

Dance, C. and Galvani, S. (2014) 'Substance use and disabilities: Experiences of adults' social care professionals and the implications for education and training.' *Social Work Education*, 33(5), pp. 670–684. DOI: 10.1080/02615479.2014.919089

Day, C., Lampraki, A., Ridings, D. and Currell, K. (2016) 'Intellectual disability and substance use/misuse: A narrative review.' *Journal of intellectual Disabilities and Offending Behaviour*, 7(1), pp. 25–34. DOI: 10.1108/JIDOB-10-2015-0041

Degenhardt, L. (2000) 'Interventions for people with alcohol use disorders and an intellectual disability: A review of the literature.' *Journal of Intellectual and Developmental Disability*, 25, pp. 135–146. DOI: 10.1080/13269780050033553

Department of Health. (DH) (2001) *Valuing People: A New Strategy for Learning Disability for the 21st Century*. A White Paper. London: The Stationery Office. Retrieved from: https://www.gov.uk/government/publications/valuing-people-a-new-strategy-for-learning-disability-for-the-21st-century [Accessed 8th March 2022]

Didden, R., Embregts, P., van der Toorn, M. and Laarhoven, N. (2009) 'Substance abuse, coping strategies, adaptive skills and behavioural and emotional problems in clients with mild to borderline intellectual disability admitted to a treatment facility: A pilot study.' *Research in Developmental Disabilities*, 30, pp. 927–932. DOI: 10.1016/j.ridd.2009.01.002.

Emerson, E., Glover, G. and Wolstenholme, J. (2014) 'Trends in age-standardised mortality rates and life expectancy of people with learning disabilities in Sheffield over a 33-year period.' *Tizard Learning Disability Review*, 19(2), pp. 90–95. DOI: 10.1108/TLDR-01-2014-0003

Emerson, E. and Hatton, C. (2013) *Health Inequalities and People with Intellectual Disabilities*. Cambridge: Cambridge University Press.

Emerson, E., Hatton, C. Robertson, J., Roberts, H., Baines, S., Evison, F. and Glover, G. (2011) *People with Learning Disabilities in England 2011*. Lancaster: Learning Disability Observatory. https://www.glh.org.uk/pdfs/PWLDAR2011.pdf [Accessed 8th March 2022].

Friedman, S. L., Helm, D. T. and Woodman, A. C. (2012) 'Unique and universal barriers: Hospice care for aging adults with intellectual disability.' *American Journal of Intellectual Development Disability*, 117(6), pp. 509–532. DOI: 10.1352/1944-7558-117.6.509

Galvani, S., Dance, C. and Wright, S. (2018) *Experiences of Hospice and Substance Use Professionals: End of Life Care for People with Alcohol and Drug Problems*. Manchester: Manchester Metropolitan University. https://endoflifecaresubstanceuse.com/wp-content/uploads/2018/11/end-of-life-care-for-people-with-substance-use-professionals-perspective-full-report.pdf [Accessed 21st March 2022].

Hammink, A. B., VanDerNagel, J. and van de Mheen, D. (2015) 'Dual disorders: Mild intellectual disability and substance abuse.' In Dom, G., Moggi, F., Dom, G. and Moggi, F. (eds.) *Co-Occurring Addictive and Psychiatric Disorders: A Practice-Based Handbook from a European Perspective*. New York: Springer-Verlag Publishing, pp. 205–220.

Heslop, P., Hoghton, M., Blair, P., Fleming, P., Marriott, A. and Russ, L. (2013) 'The need for FASTER CARE in the diagnosis of illness in people with intellectual disabilities.' *British Journal of General Practice*, 63(617), pp. 661–662. DOI: 10.3399/bjgp13X675593

Heslop, P., Blair, P. S., Fleming, P., Hoghton, M., Marriott, A. and Russ, L. (2014) 'The confidential Inquiry into premature deaths of people with intellectual disabilities in the UK: A population-based study.' *The Lancet*, 383(9920), pp. 889–895. DOI: 10.1016/S0140-6736(13)62026-7

Kepper, A., Monshouwer, K., Dorsselaer, S. V. and Vollebergh, W. (2011) 'Substance use by adolescence in special education and residential youth care institutions.' *European Child and Adolescent Psychiatry*, 20, pp. 311–319. DOI: 10.1007/s00787-011-0176-2

King, B. H., Toth, K. E., Hodapp, R. M. and Dykens, E. M. (2009) 'Intellectual disability.' In Sadock, B. J., Saock, V. A. and Ruiz, P. (eds) *Comprehensive Textbook of Psychiatry* (9th ed.). Philadelphia: Lippincott Williams & Wilkins, pp. 3444–3474.

Levin, S., Sinclair, S., Veniegas, R. and Taylor, P. (2002) 'Perceived discrimination in the context of multiple group membership.' *Psychological Science*, 13(6), pp. 557–560. DOI: 10.1111/1467-9280.00498

Livingston, J. D., Milne, T., Fang, M. L. and Amari, E. (2011) 'The effectiveness of interventions for reducing stigma related to substance use disorders: A systematic review.' *Addiction*, 107, pp. 39–50. DOI: 10.1111/j.1360-0443.2011.03601.x

Maulik, P. K., Mascarenhas, M. N., Mathers, C. D., Dua, T. and Saxena, S. (2011) 'Prevalence of intellectual disability: A meta-analysis of population-based studies.' *Research Development Disability*, 32(2), pp. 419–436. DOI: 10.1016/j.ridd.2010.12.018

McCarthy, M., Hunt, S. and Milne-Skillman, K. (2016) 'I know it was every week, but I can't be sure if it was every day: Domestic violence and women with learning disabilities.' *Journal of Applied Research in Intellectual Disabilities*, 30(2), pp. 269–282. DOI: 10.1111/jar.12237

McGillicuddy, N. B. (2006) 'A review of substance use research among those with mental retardation.' *Mental Retardation Developmental Disabilities Research Reviews*, 12, pp. 41–47. DOI: 10.1002/mrdd.20092

McKibben, L., Brazil, K., McLaughlin, D. and Hudson, P. (2020) 'Determining the informational needs of family caregivers of people with intellectual disability who require palliative care: A qualitative study.' *Palliative and Supportive Care*, 19(4), pp. 405–414. DOI: 10.1017/S1478951520001157

McLaughlin, D., Barr, O. and McIlfatrick, S. (2009) 'Delivering palliative care to those with a learning disability.' *European Journal of Palliative Care*, 16(6), pp. 302–305. http://www.jesp.eu.com/ejpc/ejpcIssue.asp?Z=93487&IssueID=100

McLaughlin, D., Barr, O., McIlfatrick, S. and McConkey, R. (2014) 'Developing a best practice model for partnership practice between specialist palliative care and intellectual disability services: A mixed methods study.' *Journal of Palliative Medicine*, 28(10), pp. 1213–1221. DOI: 10.1177/02692 16314 550373

Pelleboer-Gunnink, H. A., Van Oojouw, W. M. W., Van Weeghel, J. and Embregts, P. J. C. M. (2017) 'Mainstream health professionals' stigmatising attitudes towards people with intellectual disabilities: A systematic review.' *Journal of Intellectual Disability*, 61(5), pp. 411–434. DOI: 10.1111/jir.12353

Power, A. and Bartlett, R. (2019) 'Ageing with a learning disability: Care and support in the context of austerity.' *Social Science & Medicine*, 231, pp. 55–61 DOI: 10.1016/j.socscimed.2018.03.028.

Public Health England. (2016) *Substance Misuse in People with Learning Disabilities: Reasonable Adjustments Guidance.* https://www.gov.uk/government/publications/-substance-misuse-and-people-with-learning-disabilities/substance-misuse-in-people-with-learning-disabilities-reasonable-adjustments-guidance [Accessed 27th April 2021].

Read, S. (2013) 'Palliative care for people with intellectual disabilities: Pitfalls and potential.' *Palliative Medicine*, 27(1), pp. 3–4. DOI: 10.1177/0269216312470238

Ryan, K., Guerin, S. and McEvoy, J. (2016) 'The nature and importance of quality of therapeutic relationships in the delivery of palliative care to people with intellectual disabilities.' *BMJ Supportive & Palliative Care*, 6, pp. 430–436. DOI: 10.1136/bmjspcare-2013-000619

Taggart, L., McLaughlin, D., Quinn, B. and Milligan, V. (2006) 'An exploration of substance misuse in people with intellectual disabilities.' *Journal of Intellectual Disability Research*, 50, pp. 588–597. DOI: 10.1111/j.1365-2788.2006.00820.x.

To, W. T., Neirynck, S., Vanderplasschen, W., Vanheule, S. and Vandevelde, S. (2014) 'Substance use and misuse in persons with intellectual disabilities (ID): Results of a survey in ID and addiction services in Flanders.' *Research in Developmental Disabilities*, 35(1), pp. 1–9. DOI: 10.1016/j.ridd.2013.10.015

Tuffrey-Wijne, I., Bernal, J., Hubert, G., Butler, S. and Hollins, S. (2009) 'People with learning disabilities who have cancer: An ethnographic study.' *British Journal of General Practice*, 59, pp. 503–509. DOI: 10.3399/bjgp09X453413

Tuffrey-Wijne, I., McEnhill, L., Curfs, L. and Hollins, S. (2007) 'Palliative care provision for people with intellectual disabilities: Interviews with specialist palliative care professionals in London.' *Palliative Medicine*, 21, pp. 493–499. DOI: 10.1177/0269216307082019

Tuffrey-Wijne, I., McLaughlin, D., Curfs, L., Dusart, A., Hoenger, C., McEnhill, L., Read, S., Ryan, K., Satge, D., Straber, B., Westergard, B.-E. and Oliver, D. (2016) 'Defining consensus norms for palliative care of people with intellectual disabilities in Europe, using Delphi methods: A White Paper from the European Association of Palliative Care (EAPC).' *Palliative Medicine*, 30(5), pp. 446–455. DOI: 10.1177/0269216315600993

Tuffrey-Wijne, I. and Rose, T. (2017) 'Investigating the factors that affect the communication of death-related bad news to people with intellectual disabilities by staff in residential and supported living services: An interview study.' *Journal of Intellectual Disability Research*, 61(8), pp. 727–736. DOI: 10.1111/jir.12375

Voss, H., Vogel, A., Wagemans, A. M. A., Francke, A. L., Metsemakers, J. F. M., Courtens, A. M. and de Veers, A. J. E. (2020) 'What is important for advance care planning in the palliative phase of people with intellectual disabilities? A multi-perspective interview study.' *Journal of Applied Research in Intellectual Disability*, 33, pp. 160–171. DOI: 10.1111/jar.12653

Vrijmoeth, C., Echteld, M. A., Assendelft, P., Christians, M. G. M., Festen, D., van Schrojenstein Lantman-de Valk, H. M. J., Vissers, K. and Groot, M. (2018a) 'Development and applicability of a tool for identification of people with intellectual disabilities in need of palliative care (PALLI).' *Journal of Applied Research in Intellectual Disabilities*, 31(6), pp. 1122–1132. DOI: 10.1111/jar.12472

Vrijmoeth, C., Groot, C. M., Christians, M. G. M., Assendelft, W. J. J., Festen, D. A. M., van der Rijt, C. C. D., van Schrojenstein Lantman-de Valk, H. M. J., Vissers, K. C. P. and Echteld, M. A. (2018b) 'Feasibility and validity of a tool for identification of people with intellectual disabilities in need of palliative care (PALLI).' *Research in Developmental Disabilities*, 72, pp. 67–78. DOI: 10.1016/j.ridd.2017.10.020.

Watson, J., Wilson, E. and Hagiliassis, N. (2017) 'Supporting end of life decision making: Case studies of relational closeness in supported decision making for people with severe or profound intellectual disability.' *Journal of Applied Research in Intellectual Disabilities*, 30(6), pp. 1022–1034. DOI: 10.1111/jar.12393.

Yarwood, G., Wright, S., Templeton, L. and Galvani, S. (2018) *Experiences of Families, Friends, Carers: Phase 2 End of Life Care for People with Alcohol and Drug Problems.* Manchester: Manchester Metropolitan University. https://endoflifecaresubstanceuse.com/wp-content/uploads/2018/11/end-of-life-care-for-people-with-substance-use-family-report-phase-2-final-full-report1.pdf [Accessed 21st March 2022].

7 Improving end-of-life care for people with co-existing mental health and substance use

Lucy Webb

Introduction

People who use alcohol or other drugs problematically often have mental health co-morbidities and associated physical health and social problems that present as multiple disadvantage to services (PHE, 2017). While it is neither useful nor easy to determine direction of causality of co-morbidities, co-existing mental ill health and substance use are commonly associated with poor physical health, homelessness, frequent use of emergency services and imprisonment (PHE, 2017).

'Co-existing' or 'dual diagnosis' are the terms often used to describe a cohort of people who use drugs and/or alcohol problematically and have severe psychotic mental illnesses such as schizophrenia and bi-polar disorder, severe depression, or schizotypal or delusional disorder (NICE, 2019). The UK Department of Health/Offender Health (2009) suggests four categories of dual diagnosis:

1 Someone with a mental illness who uses substances to self-medicate, i.e. using opiates to control hallucinations in schizophrenia
2 Someone using substances that cause a mental illness, such as cannabis psychosis or crack psychosis, or mental illness caused by withdrawing from substances, such as depression following crack or amphetamine use withdrawal, or the emergence of a mental illness that has been previously 'managed' by substance use that is withdrawn, i.e. hallucinations returning when opiate use is stopped
3 Someone who has a mental illness that is worsened by substance use, even though this might offer short term relief, such as using alcohol to reduce or control anxiety
4 Someone who uses substances and has a mental illness without the two issues being related.

This typology aims to define dual diagnosis, perhaps for diagnostic purposes, however, this may further stigmatise people with multiple problems, and does not address the wider experiences of people beyond diagnosable labels (Drugscope, 2015). The National Institute for Health and Care Excellence guidelines for co-existing substance use and mental illness (NICE, 2019) seek to ensure that both

DOI: 10.4324/9781003187882-9

conditions are addressed together through joint-working and co-ordinated care, avoiding exclusion from any service because of the presence of either a mental illness or problem substance use (a 'no wrong door' policy). Currently, treatment delivery models are often based on localised arrangements for shared or integrated care depending on available expertise, with sequential treatment (one problem at a time) not recommended (CGDMD Independent Expert Working Group, 2017). This may go some way to addressing treatment access, but there are still multiple barriers to treatment due to the historical nature of having separate services, and service users' reluctance to engage due to previous negative experiences (Black, 2021).

This chapter will explore the current problems of access to end-of-life care for people with co-existing problems, and examine evidence of end-of-life care for mental health and substance use patients separately to examine what can be learnt from these individual service challenges. It will also offer a critique of current service provision, identifying the key strategies that are likely to offer a way forward to improving access.

Background

Estimates of incidence of co-morbidity vary, but this may be a product of the narrow medical definition. Most diagnostic, prevalence and incidence measures, as suggested above from the Department of Health, may only include people with severe mental illnesses such as schizophrenia and bi-polar disorder (Abou-Saleh, 2004; NICE, 2019). If wider definitions that include complex trauma (personality disorder), generalised anxiety and depression are taken into account, some estimate approximately 30%–50% of people with problematic substance use globally also have a diagnosis of mental illness (Hall et al., 2009; Lai et al., 2015; Torrens et al., 2015). This may be as high as 70% among drug users and 86% among problem alcohol users if measured more inclusively (Weaver et al., 2003; Delgado et al., 2012). Bramley and Fitzpatrick (2015) report that, among people with intersecting disadvantages (i.e. substance use, homelessness, criminal justice involvement), rates of diagnosed mental illnesses are estimated around 42%–55% but this rises to approximately 80%–92% among those who self-report a mental illness that causes them significant problems.

Indeed, people with co-existing problems may have intersecting social disadvantage *because* of the social dislocation multiple problems may represent (Fitzpatrick & Stephens, 2014), and subsequently face stigma and problems accessing services (Drinkwater et al., 2015). This group, especially those with severe multiple disadvantage (three or more disadvantages), also has low social capital; mainly relying on friends or social workers when in crisis, rather than family members (Bramley and Fitzpatrick, 2015).

This population group already has difficulty accessing mainstream services due to multiple disadvantage (Fitzpatrick et al., 2012; CFE Research and The University of Sheffield, 2020). This is not just for practical reasons, such as homeless people having no permanent address, but for cumulative problems associated with perceived discrimination from services, inability to navigate complex care pathways, and an expectation that services are 'not for them' (Making Every Adult Matter Coalition/Clinks et al., 2015; Galvani, 2018). This is compounded by underlying problems that present barriers to engaging in services. For instance, homelessness, substance use and mental illness are all associated with past experiences of childhood trauma leading to a distrust and reluctance to accept support (Magwood et al., 2019). Fond et al. (2019) indicate that people with schizophrenia and terminal cancer in France are more likely to receive a late diagnosis due to diagnostic overshadowing (attributing physical symptoms to the mental illness) and are also likely to refuse treatment because of paranoid delusions or mistrust. This is also reported globally by Park et al. (2020) and Baruth et al. (2020).

A vignette from practice illustrates the issue:

> A woman in her late 50s presented to Accident and Emergency (A&E) with stomach pains and complaining of having insects crawling over her. She was known to mental health services, having a diagnosis of schizophrenia and personality disorder, and was a heavy drinker and smoker. Typically, she lived in a variety of hostel accommodations, but frequently moved on as her smoking behaviour became an unacceptable fire risk. She often arrived at various health and social care services without appointment, with a list of complaints associated with her income support, housing, medications, and a variety of illnesses. In A&E, her stomach pains were initially dismissed as 'attention-seeking' and the insects regarded as a sensory hallucination, until it was noticed she had alcohol withdrawal symptoms and the 'insects' was a sign of delirium tremens. After admission, a series of tests identified late-stage bowel cancer.

A common problem for people with multiple disadvantage is the stigma attached to the mental illness, the substance use and the additional or consequential issues of homelessness or criminality. For this woman, stigma resulted in her behaviour being seen as attention-seeking, and her delirium tremens as a part of her schizophrenia. It was her other withdrawal symptom (severe tremor) that meant she needed to be admitted for treatment for alcohol withdrawal.

Treatment access problems for end-of-life care, however, are likely to lie further up the chain of service planning and commissioning than service provision itself. Cancers are by far the most common disease types featured in hospice referrals (Hospice UK, 2016), and there is unequal access to end-of-life care for people with conditions that commonly occur with substance misuse such as liver disease and chronic obstructive pulmonary disease (COPD) (Webb et al., 2018). However, this may be because such diseases have unpredictable prognoses, and are more difficult to manage in the hospice environment (Cox-North et al., 2013; Kendrick, 2013; Higginson et al., 2017). Pain management can require complex care for those with a history of using opiates or requiring opiate substitution therapy, or for people who have cognitive impairments due to heavy alcohol use or repeated overdose (Witham et al., 2019). Also, there may be staff training and education needs in managing patients who have difficulty in discussing end of life (Ebenau et al., 2019). Problems with end-of-life care access and quality care for people with co-existing and multiple problems are, therefore, variously identified as stemming from both the individuals themselves showing reluctance to engage, and from the services who fail to identify health problems or present clinical barriers to access.

This is also reflected in the evidence on end-of-life care for people with severe and persistent mental illnesses. Late diagnosis leaves less time to get to know the patient and build trust, or involve families in care (Fond et al. 2019; Baruth et al., 2020). Cognitive difficulties can also result in problems with involvement in decision-making about care and making advance directives (McNamara et al., 2018; Baruth et al., 2020). This is also likely to present difficulties for patients with alcohol-related brain damage such as Wernicke-Korsakoff syndrome (Alzheimer's Society, n.d.), and opiate users with cognitive impairments from repeated overdose hypoxia (O'Brien & Todd, 2009). Limited involvement of people in decisions about their care can lead to the continuation of invasive treatments and unnecessary interventions (Baruth et al., 2020), but also complicates processes for gaining informed consent. In the UK, as in most countries, legal mental capacity to consent to treatment does not rely on diagnosis but on the person's ability to understand the information given and the consequences of decision-making. This is separate from treatment for a mental illness without consent, which is governed in England and Wales by the Mental Health Act (1983). Staff without experience of mental health care may need to navigate complex issues of capacity to consent to treatment for a physical illness, when at the same time consent is not required for administering anti-psychotic medication for someone under a treatment section of the Mental Health Act (McNamara et al., 2018; McKillip et al., 2019).

Interactions with existing psychotropic medication can also be a concern for end-of-life service staff. Some antipsychotics, such as clozapine, can produce severe side effects when combined with other medication and so this treatment may be reduced. It is not uncommon therefore for psychotic symptoms to worsen during end-of-life care (McKillip et al., 2019), and emerging symptoms of psychosis may go unrecognised or be interpreted as terminal delirium (McNamara et al., 2018; Park et al., 2020). Alcohol dependence also presents medication challenges as benzodiazepines to treat alcohol withdrawal are contraindicated for liver failure, and these are the same medications used for terminal agitation. As symptom control is the key medication goal in end-of-life care, staff may also need to navigate decisions around abstinence or controlled usage (McCormac, 2017).

End-of-life care services face challenges in managing complexity presented by those living with multiple disadvantages. Staff can feel unqualified to manage patients with mental health or substance use problems, especially with those patients who lack insight. Staff may have anxieties that discussions about death may de-stabilise such patients (McNamara et al., 2018). As one of McNamara et al.'s informants suggests, these patients go in the 'too hard basket' (McNamara et al., 2018, p5). Nurses are reported to find patients 'difficult' who have multiple physical, social and cultural problems, who are non-compliant with treatment, or have challenging relatives (Ingebretsen and Sagbakken, 2016; Hawking et al., 2017; Dobrina et al., 2020). People with substance use and/or severe mental health histories often bring challenging family dynamics (Bushfield & De Ford, 2009) because of the long history of family tensions and breakdown of relationships, or they may have no family members who can be involved in their care. This means that they will lack the informal social support and involvement that end-of-life care services are familiar with (McNamara et al., 2018). It is also suggested that, in community end-of-life care, there may be concerns about public safety when prescribing opiates to people using drugs in case they are diverted for street use (Mundt-Leach, 2016).

A key issue for many commentators and practitioners, however, is the division between end-of-life care providers and treatment providers from addiction and psychiatric services. This division is argued to stem from the curative philosophy that underpins medical treatment services. The palliative approach aims to reduce symptoms and improve quality of life and is often at odds with the curative treatment goals of somatic and psychiatric medicine (McNamara et al., 2018; Sheriden, 2019). Strand et al. (2020) suggest that the 'need to treat' in psychiatric case management overrides considerations of the palliative approach, indeed, the curative philosophy and risk aversion in psychiatry may fuel the drive to minimise risk of death. However, Strand et al. (2020) suggest, that moves away from the medical curative approach in psychiatry, towards a more person-centred recovery approach that targets quality of life rather than control of symptoms, may present a gateway towards more palliative thinking in psychiatric goal-setting.

Late detection of end-of-life care needs presents a barrier to receiving timely care that enables services the space to address the complex psychosocial needs for this population. As described earlier, patients' lack of trust of services, cognitive impairments, complex family dynamics and poor social support require time and relationship-building to deliver optimum end-of-life care. Late identification is, however, an upstream problem, located more at policy and service planning level. Substance use services are now structured to focus on recovery-oriented care, targeting reduction of use and corralling social and economic support to scaffold behaviour change. Substance use practitioners subsequently fail to identify end-of-life needs (Mundt-Leach, 2016), and practitioners working with severely mentally ill people also do not refer patients to end-of-life services until late in disease progression (Fond et al., 2019). This may often be due to mistaking the signs of disease as symptoms of mental illness (McNamara et al., 2018).

Needs identified

A range of needs and strategies has been identified to improve quality of care for people with severe or enduring mental illnesses, and we can explore how these may apply equally or with adaptation to people with co-existing mental illness and substance use. Much of the existing evidence and practice recommendations also take into account the multiple disadvantages that often accompany someone with serious mental illness, therefore recommendations for improved practice are likely to apply to people living with co-existing mental illness, substance use and multiple disadvantages.

Early detection and referral

Early referral should be straightforward as the patients are often already linked into some form of social or health support. They may have key workers or contacts from social care or housing, community mental health, substance use or homeless support, and there may be regular and ongoing contacts within their formal and informal networks. These patients themselves may not, however, be personally proactive in seeking help for reasons of distrust of new services, or of people they do not already work with. Family and friends may be similarly reluctant to assist them to self-refer to services, even where patients have good relationships with concerned significant others. Clearly, early detection relies on the ability of practitioners within existing networks to identify changes in the person's health and wellbeing and facilitate diagnosis and referral. These practitioners are likely to be best placed to assist in referral especially if they have an established and trusted relationship with the person and referral pathways exist between services.

Capacity-building

The barriers to early referral appear to be that these well-placed practitioners do not have the skills or therapeutic philosophy to recognise and act on their patients' changes in health. Capacity-building in both staff training and referral pathways is suggested (McNamara et al., 2018), but this should go beyond awareness-raising. There is an increasing availability of online resources provided by the voluntary and education sector for specific end-of-life training (for example, St Mungo's, 2021) which may go some way to filling a skills gap. Clinical end-of-life staff may feel they lack skills in mental health care, but it is suggested that these skills would benefit any patient entering palliative care (Park et al., 2020). Skills such as brief cognitive behaviour therapy can be part of the psychosocial care for patients and enable staff to better respond to anxieties and depressions that commonly occur for people coming to terms with an end-of-life diagnosis.

Practitioners working with people who use substances are already coming to terms with working with an older client group. Age-sensitive treatment within substance use provision includes dealing with co-morbid conditions and having referral protocols to primary and secondary services such as general practitioners and geriatric services (Rao et al., 2018). This way of working sets a template for working with other agencies in shared or integrated care. Conversely, end-of-life services may need to better accommodate younger people, as rates of liver failure increase among younger drinkers (British Liver Trust, 2019).

Working with the multi-disciplinary team and other agencies

The complexity of end-of-life care for this population means that it would be too much to expect end-of-life care services to meet all the multiply disadvantaged patient's needs. Collaboration approaches are necessary in order to manage different aspects of a person's care; from managing anti-psychotic or opiate substitution medication to psychosocial collaboration involving the trusted significant others in the person's life. McNamara et al. (2018) stress the benefits of having multiple routes to different providers and care co-ordination to accommodate the complex needs that may be presented, including homeless shelters, A&E departments, psychiatric services and general medical wards. Relyea et al. (2019) also underline the importance of working with informal carers, often as proxy decision-makers and advocates when mental capacity is impaired. These informal carers may be family members, key workers or friends. Involving key workers from other services in the end-of-life care of patients helps overcome any mistrust of new services and unfamiliar settings. Doukas (2014) also suggests that being referred to a new service means a loss of trusted practitioners and routines for the patient, therefore having continued contact with key workers, or having these key workers acting as care co-ordinators, maintains these familiar connections. For Relyea et al. (2019), this also reassures family members who have been involved in care and who may also be mistrustful of engaging with a new service; the familiar community psychiatric nurse or recovery champion can act as an advocate and go-between.

While training staff to recognise and refer clients is recommended, end-of-life care staff may also benefit from specialist support in understanding mental illness and substance use (McNamara et al., 2018; Relyea et al., 2019). End-of-life care staff are usually familiar with managing depression, anxiety and grief in their care role, but encountering psychosis and delusions can be more challenging. The presence of unusual beliefs is common among patients with severe and enduring mental illnesses such as schizophrenia, and this element of a person's presentation is likely to be present regardless of symptom control. A delusion is part of the person's self to be accommodated in person-centred care as illustrated in the clinical example below:

> A man in his forties was referred to substance use services by the hospital ward where he was being treated for an injection site abscess. He was willing to be referred for his opiate dependency and be treated with substitution methadone, however, he was reluctant to visit the service clinic as there would be IRA (Irish Republican Army) spies there looking for him. He was convinced that the IRA was intent on hunting him down as he had been a British soldier in Northern Ireland in his youth. He had a recent history of mental illness and had been treated in the past for auditory hallucinations which he now controlled by using heroin. He agreed to be seen in the hospital outpatient clinic as the IRA would not be looking for him there.

By seeing this client in the outpatient clinic, the fixed persecutory delusion was simply accommodated as part of this man's beliefs and values rather than being challenged and viewed as a disease process to be reduced.

In discussing integrated care, Park et al. (2020) suggest that the skill set of palliative practitioners in delivering holistic care supports the integration of beliefs and psychosocial-cultural norms for their clients. They argue that the mental, psychological, spiritual and physical aspects of care could facilitate care regardless of diagnosis. Indeed, the label 'dual diagnosis' is an artifice in holistic care in which the difference between a delusion or, say, a religious belief is only relevant in navigating treatment pathways, and not relevant to holistic care. As Park et al. usefully suggest, it is not helpful to fixate on the diagnosis.

Embracing the setting: what is 'home'

As a quality outcome for end-of-life care is 'choice of place of death' (Department of Health, 2008) the setting of care for this patient group also needs to be considered. In comparison with the majority of end-of-life care service users, these patients have a wide range of settings, albeit unconventional, that may be regarded as 'home'. Practitioners still need to consider how that choice of setting for people with unstable housing can be personalised. Such settings are likely to include hostels or long-term care homes, assisted living facilities, offender rehabilitation hostels or group homes, homeless shelters, other temporary accommodation such as a friend's house or even in the street. It should also be considered that care staff may be delivering palliative care in forensic psychiatry settings or prisons. It may not be possible to support a 'home' death for many clinical, legal or practical reasons, but a goal is likely to be facilitating choice within the confines of what is do-able. Good quality end-of-life care should be delivered in any type of setting (CQC, 2016) but will require collaborative working with the staff or informal carers within that setting, and other care delivery practitioners such as mental health and substance use teams (Relyea et al., 2019). Mundt-Leach (2016) indicates that what a person in need of care means by 'home' may be where there are trusted people and familiar surroundings, and this is likely to apply to their family or friends too.

Challenging presentations: behaviour and lack of insight or capacity

The practicalities of multiple medication regimes, communication barriers and cognitive impairments can present end-of-life care practitioners with treatment and care challenges (McKillip et al., 2019). Consent and capacity issues need to be separated from any diagnosis of mental illness, and taken with clear reference to capacity guidelines. If a patient can understand information given, can understand the consequences of their care decision, and can communicate their wishes, then any apparent unwise decision needs to be respected (Office of the Public Guardian, 2007). This principle of unwise decision-making is likely to apply to fixed delusions held by a person (as the vignette above describes), but if a temporary mental illness symptom interferes with capacity, such as deeply depressive thinking associated with clinical depression, then this may indicate lack of capacity. An important element of the Mental Health Act in England and Wales (Mental Health Act, 1983), however, is that any treatment under the Act can only be for a mental illness, and does not apply to substance dependency. Therefore, a person without capacity due to cognitive impairment can receive end-of-life care under the Mental Capacity Act of 2005 (Mental

Capacity Act, 2005) if it is deemed in their best interests, but not by invoking the Mental Health Act.

Lack of insight does not necessarily require a mental illness, nor denote a cognitive impairment. However, some patients with severe mental illness that is refractory (unresponsive to treatment) can result in lack of insight into both their condition and impending death. This is not wholly uncommon for patients with paranoid schizophrenia, bi-polar disorder, some personality disorders or even severe anorexia nervosa (Strand et al., 2020). Some patients may struggle to understand their terminal diagnosis, or refuse curative treatment, resulting in end-stage conditions. While this may be difficult for care staff to understand, clearly the palliative approach is for symptom reduction and aiding the person to have good quality of life (Baruth et al., 2020). Decorte et al. (2020) discuss a holistic approach to end-of-life care, the Oyster Care model, for people with an inability to understand and comply with their care. The Oyster Care model is being developed in Belgium to improve end-of-life care for patients with untreatable cognitive, behavioural and social challenges. These clients are likely to be in specialist residential or forensic care rather than end-of-life care settings, but still require good quality palliative care from their care staff. The model focusses specifically on quality of life and prompts a therapeutic environment that shields patients from suffering physically, mentally, socially and existentially, while aiming to preserve dignity. There is an emphasis on creative therapies and a reduction of diagnosis-driven care planning or attempts to improve insight or decision-making. Oyster Care was created in response to the national legalisation of euthanasia in Belgium and the introduction of recovery-oriented approaches in psychiatry. It offers quality of life alternatives to curative treatment for severely mentally ill patients so that good quality terminal care is delivered with dignity.

Inclusive models of care

Much of the available evidence indicates a need for inclusive models of care which adopt a form of shared care, integrated care or joint working between services, which is inclusive of existing informal support. The fragmentation and specialism of health and social care services presents problems for shared and integrated care towards the end of life (Sheriden, 2019). Divisions between primary and secondary care, and localised non-governmental organisation (NGO) specialist care, force a reliance on establishing local connections and referral pathways to co-ordinate care, but provides little incentive for organised shared care arrangements. It is current policy for people with co-morbid needs in the community to receive shared care, with mental health services acting as lead organisations for treatment (NICE, 2016), but this way of working may still be facing problems through lack of mental health service resources (Parliamentary & Health Service Ombudsman, 2018), and has not yet been translated to inpatient end-of-life care in hospitals, care homes or specialist hospice settings. As applies in the principle of a duty of care, whichever service has responsibility for the person in situ, has, in the first instance, overall responsibility for care. End-of-life care already provides a holistic care template that could provide a platform for integrating care, but mental health services currently lead on curative care of patients with co-existing disorders. The current model of 'no wrong door' access to care for people with co-existing disorders suggests an approach for those multiply disadvantaged to access end-of-life care. Integrated care for this patient group perhaps could be determined by predominant care needs or who picks up the issue first. End-of-life care services are already open to holistic, biopsychosocial-spiritual models and may be the best default lead service. However, they need the training and resource capacity take this lead.

Evidence of current practice indicates that end-of-life care services tend to rely on staff establishing multi-disciplinary working relationships themselves (Park et al., 2020). Case conferencing that includes informal carers is found to be important, not just for gaining more insight into the person's needs but also in appreciating what informal carers need (McNamara et al., 2018), and working with the informal carer as the patient's advocate or decision-maker (Baruth et al., 2020). Regular case conferencing with mental health case workers and a primary care representative is recommended, along with establishing a lead team member or organisation, depending on the relative dominance of the patient's symptoms (McNamara et al., 2018).

There is a danger however, that care could become medicalised or impersonal in a systematised care package. While there is a need for specialist input, for example, regarding anti-psychotic medication, for Park et al. (2020), keeping a focus on holistic and reflexive personal care is most important. Their informants suggested a need for embedded mental health specialists within their team. The authors indicate a '*consultative versus integrative*' system dichotomy between having specialists to consult or having expertise within the system (Park et al., 2020, p5). Practitioner informants from end-of-life care appeared to value whatever model best supports holistic care. Either way, what appears to be valued is interdisciplinary education and the availability of practice skills in mental health and substance use from which to learn.

The need to respond to the ageing population of people engaging with substance use services may indicate one way forward in at least addressing late presentation and diagnosis. As Rao et al. (2019) suggest, substance use services should establish links with primary and secondary care and NGO services to address chronic physical health needs for their patients, and this suggests a health and social care systems approach to tackling co-morbidities. An improved awareness of health and social needs for older substance users among service staff, with developed care pathways and shared or integrated care, can also break down the barriers of silo working. Additionally, the growing awareness of the need for end-of-life care services to provide for more managerially challenging conditions such as liver disease and COPD (Kendrick, 2013; Higginson et al. 2017) highlights the need to improve access for substance users. Integrated care pathways and joint working may better address clinical management issues for end-of-life services and provide referral pathways for patients with end-of-life care needs – including housing, substance use and mental health services (Fitzpatrick et al., 2012).

Conclusion

The difficulties experienced by mental health, substance use and end-of-life care services in meeting the needs of patients with co-existing substance and mental health issues indicates need for an expansion of policy. Currently care policies for this group focus on recovery and community aid. There is no recognition of palliative approaches in substance use services and little recognition in mental health services. The onus for change may be more on mental health and substance use services to develop skills and care philosophies that encompass chronic co-morbidities among older service users and to develop referral pathways at least to end the problem of late diagnosis of a life-limiting illness. A move towards a palliative care model in psychiatry that adopts the symptom reduction and quality of life goals may be a start in changing thinking.

References

Abou-Saleh, M. (2004) 'Dual diagnosis: Management within a psychosocial context.' *Advances in Psychiatric Treatment*, 10(5), pp. 352–360. DOI: 10.1192/apt.10.5.352

Alzheimer's Society. (no date) *Wernicke-Korsakoff Syndrome*. https://www.alzheimers.org.uk/about-dementia/types-dementia/wernicke-korsakoff-syndrome

Baruth, J., Ho, J., Mohammad, S., and Lapid, M. (2020) 'End-of-life care in schizophrenia: A systematic review.' *International Psychogeriatrics*. DOI: 10.1017/S1041610220000915

Black, L.-A. (2021) *Mental ill health and substance misuse: Dual Diagnosis*. Research and Information Service Research Paper No 19/21, Northern Ireland Assembly.

Bramley, G., and Fitzpatrick, S., (2015) *Hard edges: Mapping severe and multiple disadvantage*. London. Langley Chase Foundation. http://www.lankellychase.org.uk/our_work/policy_research/hard_edges

British Liver Trust. (2019) *The alarming impact of liver disease in the UK Facts and statistics*. Bournemouth: British Liver Trust. Available at: https://britishlivertrust.org.uk/about-us/media-centre/statistics/

Bushfield, S., and De Ford, B. (2009) *End of life care and addiction: A family systems approach*. New York: Springer.

CFE Research and The University of Sheffield. (2020) *Improving access to mental health support for people experiencing multiple disadvantage*. London: The National Lottery Community Fund. Available at: https://issuu.com/voicesofstoke/docs/report-summary-improving-access-to-mental-health-s

CGDMD Independent Expert Working Group. (2017). *Drug misuse and dependence: UK guidelines on clinical management*. London: Clinical Guidelines on Drug Misuse and Dependence.

Cox-North, P., Doorenbos, A., Shannon, S., Scott, J., and Curtis, J. (2013) 'The transition to end-of-life care in end-stage liver disease.' *Journal of Hospice and Palliative Nursing*, 15(4), pp. 209–215. DOI: 10.1097/NJH.0b013e318289f4b0

CQC. (2016) *A different ending: Addressing inequalities in end of life care*. Newcastle Upon Tyne: Care Quality Commission.

Department of Health. (2002) *Mental health policy and implementation guide – Dual diagnosis good practice guide*. London: Department of Health.

Department of Health. (2008) *End of life care strategy promoting high quality care for all adults at the end of life*. London: Department of Health.

Department of Health/Offender Health. (2009) *A guide for the management of dual diagnosis in prisons.* London: DH/Offender Health.

Dobrina, R., Chialchia, S., and Palese, A. (2020) '"Difficult patients" in the advanced stages of cancer as experienced by nursing staff: A descriptive qualitative study.' *European Journal of Oncology Nursing*, 46. DOI: 10.1016/j.ejon.2020.101766

Doukas, N. (2014) 'Are methadone counselors properly equipped to meet the palliative care needs of older adults in methadone maintenance treatment? Implications for training.' *Journal of Social Work in End-Of-Life and Palliative Care*, 10(2), pp. 186–204. DOI: 10.1080/15524256.2014.906370

Drinkwater, N., Graham, J., Kempster, A., Thomas, S., and Making Every Adult Matter Policy Management Group. (2015) *Solutions from the Frontline: Recommendations or Policymakers on Supporting People with Multiple Needs.* Making Every Adult Matter Coalition, Clink, Homeless Link, Mind; Lankelly Chase Foundation. Available online at: http://www.meam.org.uk/wp-content/uploads/2018/09/Solutions-from-the-Frontline-WEB.pdf

Drugscope. (2015). *Mental health and substance use.* London: Drugscope. Available at: https://drugscope.blogspot.com/2015/01/briefing-mental-health-and-substance.html

Ebenau, A., Dijkstra, B., Huurne, C., Hasselaa, J., Vissers, K., and Groot, M. (2019) 'Palliative care for people with substance use disorder and multiple problems: A qualitative study on experiences of patients and proxies.' *BMC Palliative Care*, 18, p. 56. DOI: 10.1186/s12904-019-0443-4

Fitzpatrick, S., Bramley, G., and Johnsen, S. (2012) *Multiple exclusion homelessness in the UK: An overview of findings: Briefing paper no. 1.* Multiple Exclusion Homelessness in the UK: Briefing Papers, Heriot-Watt University, Edinburgh. http://www.sbe.hw.ac.uk/research/ihurer/homelessness-social-exclusion/multipleexclusion-homelessness.htm

Fitzpatrick, S., and Stephens, M. (2014) 'Welfare regimes, social values and homelessness: Comparing responses to marginalised groups in six European countries.' *Housing Studies*, 29(2), pp. 215–234. DOI: 10.1080/02673037.2014.848265

Fond, G., Salas, S., Pauly, V., Baumstarck, K., Bernard, C., Orleans, V., Llorca, P-M., Lancon, C., Auquier, P., and Boyer, L. (2019) 'End-of-life care among patients with schizophrenia and cancer: A population-based cohort study from the French national hospital database.' *Lancet Public Health*, 4, pp. e583–e591. DOI: 10.1016/S2468-2667(19)30187-2

Galvani, S. (2018) *End of life care for people with alcohol and other drug problems: What we know and what we need to know. Final Project Report.* Manchester: Manchester Metropolitan University. Available online at: http://e-space.mmu. ac.uk/622052/1/EOLC%20Final%20 overview%20 report%2027%20November%202018%20 PRINT%20VERSION.pdf.

Hall, W., Degenhardt, L., and Teeson, M. (2009) Reprint of "Understanding comorbidity between substance use, anxiety and affective disorders: Broadening the research base." *Addictive Behavior*, 34(10), pp. 795–799. DOI: 10.1016/j.addbeh.2009.03.010

Hawking, M., Curlin, F., and Yoon, J. (2017) 'Courage and compassion: Virtues in caring for so called "difficult" patients.' *American Journal of Ethics*, 19, pp. 357–363. DOI: 10.1001/journalofethics.2017.19.4.medu2-1704

Higginson, I., Reilly, C., Bajwah, S., Maddocks, M., Constantini, M., and Gao, W. (2017) 'Which patients with advanced respiratory disease die in hospital? A 14-year population-based study of trends and associated factors.' *BMC Medicine*, 15, p. 19. DOI 10.1186/s12916-016-0776-2

Hospice UK. (2016) *National survey of patient activity data for specialist palliative care services: Minimum data set (MDS) summary report for the year 2014–15.* London: The National Council for Palliative Care.

Ingebretsen, L., and Sagbakken, M. (2016) 'Hospice nurses' emotional challenges in their encounters with the dying.' *International Journal of Qualitative Studies on Health and Wellbeing*, 11, p. 31170. DOI: 10.3402/qhw.v11.31170

Kendrick, E. (2013) *Getting it right: Improving end of life care for people living with liver disease*. London: National End of Life Care Programme. https://eprints.ncl.ac.uk/pub_details2.aspx?pub_id=191412

Lai, H., Cleary, M., Sitharthan, T., and Hunt, G. E. (2015) 'Prevalence of comorbid substance use, anxiety and mood disorders in epidemiological surveys, 1990–2014: A systematic review and meta-analysis.' *Drug and Alcohol Dependence*, 154, pp. 1–13. DOI: 10.1016/j.drugalcdep.2015.05.031

Magwood, O., Leki, V. Y., Kpade, V., Saad, A., Alkhateeb, Q., Gebremeskel, A., Rehman, A., Hannigan, T., Pinto, N., Sun, A. H., Kendall, C., Kozloff, N., Tweed, E. J., Ponka, D., and Pottie, K. (2019) 'Common trust and personal safety issues: A systematic review on the acceptability of health and social interventions for persons with lived experience of homelessness.' *PLoS One*, 14(12), p. e0226306. DOI: 10.1371/journal.pone.0226306

Making Every Adult Matter Coalition/Clinks, DrugScope, Homeless Link and Mind. (2015) *Voices from the frontline: Listening to people with multiple needs, and those who support them*. London: Lankelly Chase Foundation.

McCormac, A. (2017) 'Alcohol dependence in palliative care: A review of the current literature.' *Journal of Palliative Care*, 32(3–4), pp. 108–112. DOI: 10.1177/0825859717738445

McKillip, K., Lott, A., and Swetz, K. (2019) 'Respecting autonomy and promoting the patient's good in the setting of serious terminal and concurrent mental illness.' *Yale Journal of Biology and Medicine*, 92, pp. 597–602. PMCID: PMC6913820

McNamara, B., Same, A., Rosenwax, L., and Kelly, B. (2018) 'Palliative care for people with schizophrenia: A qualitative study of an under-serviced group in need.' *BMC Palliative Care*, 17, p. 53. DOI: 10.1186/s12904-018-0309-1

Mental Capacity Act 2005, C.9. (2005). London: HMSO. https://www.legislation.gov.uk/ukpga/2005/9/contents

Mental Health Act 1983, C.20. (1983). London: HMSO. https://www.legislation.gov.uk/ukpga/1983/20/contents

Mundt-Leach, R. (2016) 'End of life and palliative care of patients with drug and alcohol addiction.' *Mental Health Practice*. DOI: 10.7748/mhp.2016.e1148

NICE. (2016) *Coexisting severe mental illness and substance misuse: Community health and social care services (NG58)*. London: National Institute for Health and Care Excellence.

NICE. (2019) *Coexisting severe mental illness and substance misuse (Quality Standard 188)*. London: National Institute for Health and Care Excellence.

O'Brien, P., and Todd, J. (2009) 'Hypoxic brain injury following heroin overdose.' *Brain Impairment*, 10(2), pp. 169–179. DOI: 10.1375/brim.10.2.169

Office of the Public Guardian. (2007) *Mental capacity act 2005 code of practice*. London: The Stationery Office. ISBN 9780117037465

Park, T., Hegadoren, K., and Workun, B. (2020) 'Working at the intersection of palliative end-of-life and mental health care: Provider perspectives.' *Journal of Palliative Care*, pp. 1–7. DOI: 10.1177/0825859720951360

Parliamentary and Health Service Ombudsman. (2018) *Maintaining momentum: Driving improvements in mental health care*. H906, London: PHSO.

Public Health England (PHE). (2017) *Better care for people with co-occurring mental health and alcohol/drug use conditions. A guide for commissioners and service providers*. London: Public Health England.

Rao, R., Crome, I., Crome, P., and Iliffe, S. (2018) 'Substance misuse in later life: Challenges for primary care: A review of policy and evidence.' *Primary Health Care Research and Development*, 20(e117), pp. 1–7. DOI: 10.1017/S1463423618000440

Relyea, E., MacDonald, B., Cattaruzza, C., and Marshall, D. (2019) 'On the margins of death: A scoping review on palliative care and schizophrenia.' *Journal of Palliative Care*, 34(1), pp. 62–69. DOI: 10.3389/fpsyt.2021.752897

Sheridan, A. (2019) 'Palliative care for people with serious mental illnesses.' *Comment: The Lancet*, 4, pp. E545–e546. DOI: 10.1016/S2468-2667(19)30205-1

St Mungo's. (2021) *Palliative care*. Available at: https://www.mungos.org/service_model/palliative-care/

Strand, M., Sjostrand, M., and Lindblad, A. (2020) 'A palliative care approach in psychiatry: Clinical implications.' *BMC Medical Ethics*, pp. 21–29. DOI: 10.1186/s12910-020-00472-8

Torrens, M., Mestre-Pintó, J., Domingo-Salvany, A., and EMCDDA project group. (2015) *Comorbidity of substance use and mental disorders in Europe*. Lisbon, Portugal: European Monitoring Centre for Drugs and Drug Addiction. ISSN 2314–9264.

Weaver, T., Madden, P., Charles, V., Stimson, G., Renton, A., Tyrer, P., Barnes, T., Bench, C., Middleton, H., Wright, N., Paterson, S., Shanahan, W., Seivewright, N., Ford, C., and on behalf of the Comorbidity of Substance Misuse and Mental Illness Collaborative (COSMIC) Study Team. (2003) 'Comorbidity of substance misuse and mental illness in community mental health and substance misuse services.' *British Journal of Psychiatry*, 183, pp. 304–313. DOI: 10.1192/bjp.183.4.304. PMID: 14519608.

Webb, L., Galvani, S., and Wright, S. (2018). *Scoping review of existing database evidence: End of life care for people with alcohol and drug problems*. Manchester: Manchester Metropolitan University. https://e-space.mmu.ac.uk/620120/

Witham, G., Galvani, S., and Peacock, M. (2019) 'End of life care for people with alcohol and drug problems: Findings from a rapid evidence assessment.' *Health and Social Care in the Community*, 27, pp. e637–e650. DOI: 10.1111/hsc.12807

8   Ageing (dis)gracefully

People who inject drugs living with hepatitis C and the provision of end-of-life care

Peter Higgs

This chapter is dedicated to Jude Byrne who died on March 5, 2021 after a short stint in palliative care. Her short illness and subsequent death were during the early stages of preparing this writing. The title was hers and is based on her tireless life-long commitment to the lives of people who use drugs. Rest In Power Jude.

Introduction

The best practice provision of palliative care for older people has been identified as an important public health challenge by the World Health Organisation. However, the specific needs of older people with histories of injecting drug use are not well understood. This chapter outlines the major gaps in current knowledge of the health and well-being of older opiate users especially as it relates to the provision of end-of-life care. As outlined below, there are good reasons to expect substantial health problems (including the need for palliative care) among this population as they grow older.

Of the health conditions many people with a history of injecting drugs (opioids and/or amphetamines) encounter, the most common are blood-borne viruses (BBVs). Among them are HIV and viral hepatitis, with hepatitis C – only identified in 1989 – being the most prominent. Before then it was simply known as non-A non-B hepatitis as it was causing inflammation of the liver in people who were exposed to it (Pawlotsky et al., 2015). Since the 1970s people who inject drugs have been the population most affected by hepatitis C and are often confronted with a range of additional challenges as they grow older (Yarnell et al., 2020). There are negative health-related complications from living with hepatitis C, most commonly liver disease, but also a wide range of broader social ones. Stigma, discrimination, social isolation, economic hardship and psychological distress are all known to affect a person's quality of life at any point during their lifespan (Chang et al., 2019).

In this chapter the impact of growing older and having a history of injecting drug use is described. Specific implications for people working as practitioners as well as policy makers, in the drug and alcohol and aged care sectors, are also suggested.

DOI: 10.4324/9781003187882-10

Hepatitis C and ageing among people who inject drugs

People who inject drugs, the population most affected by hepatitis C in Australia (and most Western country settings), are often confronted with additional challenges as they age. In this chapter the focus will be on the situation in Australia, but this can be equally applied to other similar settings where people who inject drugs are part of the ageing population (Thandi and Browne, 2019).

As noted above, the hepatitis C virus infection is highly prevalent among people who inject drugs and is likely to reach saturation at around 90% prevalence in older opiate users (Hagan et al., 2007). The outcomes of hepatitis C virus infection typically manifest themselves 20–30 years after the initial exposure. Therefore, people in their 1950s, who are now included in the older person demographic and had begun injecting in their late teens, are at risk of impaired liver function and liver damage, including cirrhosis and cancer (Shepard et al., 2005). There is also evidence that hepatitis C-related morbidity and mortality can be greatly exacerbated by alcohol consumption (Niederau et al., 1998). While not a universal experience, findings from research in North America and more recently in South Africa suggest that alcohol use among people on methadone treatment increases following any decline in heroin intake (Morgan et al., 2020).

Consistent with the ageing demographic of the general Australian population (and that of many other first world countries), the proportion of older people who inject drugs is increasing as is awareness of it as a public health issue (Yarnell et al., 2020). This has been accompanied by increasing research momentum on and with older opiate users over the past decade. For example, in 2009, the Scottish Drugs Forum held a one-day conference in Glasgow, Scotland, entitled *Responding to the 'Trainspotting Generation' – An Ageing Problem*. Soon after, Harm Reduction International, one of the leading non-government organisations globally, dedicated to reducing the most harmful health, social and legal consequences of drug use and drug policy, held a plenary session at its 2010 meeting which heard first-hand a range of perspectives on the most pressing issues facing people injecting drugs and the service providers they came into contact with.

Studies identifying the specific health needs of older opiate users have been undertaken in North America (Rosenburg, 1995; Anderson and Levy, 2003; Tuchman, 2003) and the United Kingdom (Beynon et al., 2007, 2009). These data suggest that much research remains to be done especially in ways to better understand how the life trajectories of ageing and drug use co-occur within the context of different age-cohorts, and across differing life circumstances. Other studies also suggest that the natural progression of certain diseases mean that their symptoms may only manifest in older age. Therefore, the lives of older people using drugs (including those who are prescribed opiate agonist treatment) are likely to be characterised by considerable levels of morbidity (Beynon et al., 2010; Han et al., 2022). The palliative care experiences of this group of people have largely been undescribed.

However, there is longitudinal research with people using drugs from which to build an evidence base and to highlight the needs of this unique population group. Several North American and Western European natural history studies of people who inject drugs followed participants over several decades (Oppenheimer et al., 1994; Hser et al., 2007). In California, for example, researchers found at least half of the participants they interviewed (mean age at 33 years of follow-up was 54.7 years) were still using illicit opioids and almost three-quarters were either currently being treated with methadone or had been in the previous 12 months (Hser et al., 2007). A study of people who inject drugs in London indicated that the health status of those who were still using opioids after 22 years of follow-up was significantly worse than the health of those who had stopped using opioids (Tobutt et al., 1996). Sixty-five percent of those interviewed reported some physical illness which they believed was a direct result of their injecting drug use.

From these studies it is clear that there are a proportion of people who will continue to inject drugs (especially opioids) from their late teens right through their adult life and into older age. As awareness of this ageing population increases, there will need to be effective support for them and responsive palliative care programmes for people who use drugs as they age. This will become especially prominent at the end of their lives and will require services to actively involve the population most affected in the development of specific programmes to address any issues arising (Higgs et al., 2020). Despite the data from overseas and the increasing evidence in Australia, the issue of ageing, injecting drug use, living with the health consequences of hepatitis C virus and palliative care, remains an unexplored area of sensitively designed programmatic responses.

Notwithstanding the increasing diagnoses of hepatitis C virus among Australians aged over 50 years and the high proportion of people ageing with the virus, there is limited qualitative research with older people living with hepatitis C describing their social, health and support needs. Previous assessments of the needs of people living with hepatitis C virus (Australian Hepatitis Council, 2003; Richmond, 2009), have not examined the potential impact of ageing on the delivery of services or the changing needs of people living with hepatitis C as they grow older. The omission of ageing from previous Australian national strategies for hepatitis C is significant because these are pivotal documents that direct both the activities of community agencies and the framing of future government policy.

Added to this is some consistency in the determination of an age cut-off for 'old' or 'ageing' for both policy makers and researchers. This is somewhat arbitrary not least because age-related changes vary tremendously across individuals and because there is some evidence to suggest that age-related health impacts affect the body's reactions to alcohol and other drugs as early as 50 years of age (Yarnell et al., 2020).

Surveillance data from the Annual National Needle and Syringe Program Survey (ANSPS) and the Illicit Drug Reporting System (IDRS) suggest there is a large, ageing cohort of opioid injectors in Australia. Over the past 25 years (1995–2019), the proportion of respondents aged 45 years or older has increased significantly (Heard et al., 2020). More specifically, the proportion of participants aged over 45 years in the ANSPS interviews increased from less than 2% of respondents in 1995, to 42% who were aged 45 years or older in 2019. Other data corroborates this, with the mean age at interview for the IDRS surveillance system showing an increase from 29 to 44 years between 2000 and 2020, with a significant but increasing minority aged between 50 and 66 across most years (Sutherland et al., 2021). However, neither the ANSPS nor the IDRS surveillance data analyse or publish data specifically focussed on older participants recruited in these studies. Therefore, it is currently impossible to discern differences in drug use or risk behaviour patterns for older people who currently inject. Further evidence of the ageing cohort can be found in the national opiate agonist treatment data. More than 53,300 people were receiving pharmacotherapy treatment for opioid dependence on the most recent census taken in June 2020 (Australian Institute of Health and Welfare [AIHW], 2021), of which 22% were aged over 50 years of age and over 5,000 people were aged over 60 years of age. There is a large and growing population here who are likely to have substantial unmet needs as they move towards greater contact and engagement with the aged care sector.

Interviews conducted by the leading organisation representing people who use drugs, the Australian Injecting and Illicit Drug Users League (AIVL), identified that many of the people they spoke to who inject drugs did not anticipate or prepare for older age themselves, and were surprised to find themselves and their peers advancing in years. Despite the availability of effective hepatitis C treatment medications in a range of different primary and tertiary care settings, they were confronted by friends and other people who inject drugs dying of liver disease related to hepatitis C. The research interviews and the resulting discussion paper highlight a number of overarching issues for older drug injectors which are explained in some detail below (Madden and Parkes, 2010).

The issues could be summarised across seven key themes. The first of these included the direct impacts on individual health from the cumulative effect of either years of drug injecting or the continued use of opiate agonist treatment like methadone or indeed more frequently a combination of the two. Second, those interviewed identified difficulties and frustration in obtaining consistent and quality health care from the primary health services they were attending. For many this was complicated by difficulties in having their chronic pain managed – a problem which is complicated by their tolerance to opioids and health issues associated with getting older (Murphy et al., 2018). The third theme includes the impact that other social determinants included poorer socio-economic status and the disproportionate impact that the cost of pharmacotherapy treatment for heroin dependence had on disposable income (Rowe, 2008). The fourth were ongoing issues associated with living with viral hepatitis including uncertainties about the best way to manage liver health. The ongoing management of liver health has also been recently highlighted in interviews with people seeking hepatitis C treatment (Goutzamanis et al., 2018). The fifth theme identified was the burden that poor oral health had on quality of life which was also raised as an increasingly difficult problem for people to manage, not least because of the difficulty in finding affordable oral health care.

The final two themes identified by the older people interviewed have particular relevance for developing effective and responsive palliative care programmes which will be explored in more detail through this chapter. The issue relates to managing their 'dual (using and non-using) lives', especially for people who were not necessarily injecting drugs regularly. People were conscious of feeling like they were constantly negotiating with service providers including their doctors and their pharmacist. Issues of confronting stigma and discrimination were also ever present when managing relationships with family, especially adult children. The negative impact of internalised stigma and problems with normalising opiate treatment across all health care settings has been identified in more recent research with people who had been long-term consumers of methadone (Mayock and Butler, 2021).

More recently AIVL's advocacy for people injecting drugs in Australia has included noting the substantial effort required to maintain a healthy life while continuing to inject opioids. AIVL identified that older drug injectors are a population group with particular needs that are not being addressed by the health and welfare agencies with which they currently interact (Parkes, 2010). This has led to further recommendations that are directly related to the aged care sector and for those working in palliative care. This comprehensive needs analysis identifies the practitioner and system requirements for supporting healthy ageing among older people who inject drugs. It makes a number of recommendations for systemic change, including the need to build capacity among aged care services to meet the unique needs of this ageing cohort (AIVL, 2019).

Health problems for older opioid users

Data from Australian studies also suggest that older Australian opiate users will face numerous health problems as they get older. Injecting drug use is known to be associated with a wide range of potential harms and negative health sequelae, including fatal and non- fatal overdose (Dietze et al., 2005), blood-borne viral infections such as hepatitis B and C (Crofts and Aitken, 1997, Maher et al., 2006) and soft tissue and vascular problems (Dwyer et al., 2009). Many of these conditions are chronic, producing lasting ill-health for affected individuals and substantial economic costs to the public health system and the community. The management of long-term dependencies on opioids can make the recognition of life-limiting conditions difficult for people who have become familiar with negotiating the side effects of opioid withdrawal which can delay treatment seeking (Mateu-Gelabert et al., 2010; Bluthenthal et al., 2020).

Tobacco-related morbidity is also likely to be of serious concern for older opiate injectors as tobacco consumption among people who inject drugs is substantially higher than in the general population. Some studies suggest that up to 95% of their participants report smoking daily (Clarke et al., 2001). While tobacco smoking rates in the general population continue to decline, it remains concentrated in more marginalised groups such as people who inject drugs with some research suggesting older people are more interested in smoking cessation (Clarke et al., 2001).

Opioids are also thought to increase dental health problems because they can reduce the amount of saliva produced (Laslett et al., 2008). Such problems are likely to be exacerbated with continued opiate use over an extended period of time. There is also some evidence from Chicago, USA, indicating that the prevalence of injecting-related injuries like abscesses and phlebitis increases with age, making venous access to support palliative and end-of-life interventions more challenging (Anderson and

Levy, 2003). In the general population, poorer health outcomes are associated with social and economic status (Adams et al., 2009). People who inject drugs (at least the ones who participate in research) are disproportionally drawn from backgrounds with lower economic disadvantage, limited formal education and inadequate housing. These factors are all likely to contribute to increasingly poor physical and mental health for older opiate injectors. This needs to be considered in terms of the impact this will have for both palliative care and aged care service provision.

The implication, highlighted later in the chapter, is that management of pain relief will potentially be more problematic.

The challenges for practice responses

Health care providers, not just those in aged care settings, can overlook illicit drug use among older people, mistaking the symptoms for those of dementia, depression, or other problems common to older adults (Blow, 1998). Current tools used to screen for problematic drug use have not been validated for use in older populations. The Diagnostic and Statistical Manual of Mental Disorders V for substance abuse, for example, was developed and validated in young and middle-aged populations and some criteria for identifying opioid dependence, such as a reduction in physical activity, may not be appropriate for older people whose levels of activity often naturally decline as they age.

Opiate agonist treatment, primarily methadone and buprenorphine, now helps numerous Australians with heroin using histories to avoid most of the negative health consequences of opiate injecting (Mattick et al., 2008). While methadone was first prescribed in Australia in 1968, it was not made widely available until 1985. The opiate agonist treatment programme expanded dramatically in the 1990s and was enhanced in 2000 through the inclusion of buprenorphine, the combination buprenorphine /naloxone and more recently long-acting injectable buprenorphine (Salter et al., 2020). There are now more than 50,000 Australians prescribed opiate agonists by general practitioners and dosed daily in community pharmacies, about two-thirds of whom are prescribed methadone (AIHW, 2020).

A range of barriers to accessing health care for people who inject drugs have been identified, including stigma and discrimination (Stoove et al., 2005; Radcliffe and Stevens, 2008), health workers' lack of confidentiality (Ho and Maher, 2008), service models that are unacceptable or inaccessible (Winter et al., 2008; Coupland et al., 2009), cultural differences in approaches to managing health problems (Higgs et al., 2009), economic disadvantage and competing priorities (McCoy et al., 2001). Some studies have also highlighted that people who inject drugs often do not seek health care or delay accessing it (Morgan et al., 2015). This means that when people are required to make use of end-of-life care services they are doing so at a late stage of their illness.

Relatively few older adults with opiate dependencies who inject drugs appear to seek on-going primary health care, although many have regular contact with pharmacies and drug and alcohol specialists (Higgs and Dietze, 2017). Primary care and other health care services may provide a valuable opportunity to screen for any potential health problems associated with either opiate use or ageing, including diabetes, osteoporosis, arthritis or thyroid problems (Gossop and Moos, 2008; Higgs, 2015). There remain few qualitative studies in Australia that have examined barriers to health care access for older people who inject drugs especially in the context of palliative care.

It is also important to emphasise the many challenges faced by people with family and friends who end up being confronted by the aged care health system and the need for empathetic palliative care. As identified in recent work by AIVL (AIVL, 2019) both the aged care and palliative care sectors have limited previous experience in working with the population of people who inject drugs. These sectors are where the complexities of the issues for older people injecting drugs become most obvious. Added to this are issues to do with the workforce stability. Recent qualitative research has highlighted staff retention and mobility are of concern for both nursing and non-nursing staff in both community and residential care settings for the aged care sector (Xiao et al., 2021).

Case Study (composite case from the people I have worked with over the past 25 years)

Harry is a man I first met while we were doing research with younger people (aged under 30) looking to better understand the impact of street-based drugs markets and the dynamics of hepatitis C transmission among people's injecting networks. Harry, now aged in his late 1950s, has been injecting heroin on and off (mostly on) and tobacco smoking since his late teens but rarely drinks alcohol. Harry was a regular in the street-based drug market where I spent most of my research time. He had a long history of incarceration though had not been in prison for at least a decade. He tells me that his biggest 'health issue' is affordable housing and for the whole time I have known him has never had a place to call his own. He has recently taken to sleeping in the park.

Recently, Harry has attended the emergency department more regularly and is known there as a 'frequent flyer'. He is rarely admitted for longer than a few hours but has had some longer stays for what he tells me are chest infections. I know he has some family, mostly estranged, though I've never met them, and I am increasingly concerned about his deteriorating health. The last time I saw him he had just got out of hospital and told me his liver was playing up and they want him to go in for some more tests. I suspect he has advanced stage liver cancer and I encouraged him to attend the next appointment offering to go with him. At this appointment Harry got the news he perhaps had been in denial about – his liver had at least two tumours and some spread to his lungs. Things were fast coming to a head for Harry and we left this appointment with a follow up to the liver specialist and an outpatient appointment with the SMART (Symptom Management and Referral Team) Clinic established to manage early referrals.

Challenges raised by *Harry* for palliative care, the liver clinic and other staff working in drug treatment

The issue of how best to manage chronic pain, in this case liver cancer-related pain, with pharmaceutical opioids for people with long standing opiate use and tolerance created a number of tense conversations between the SMART staff and Harry's drug treatment specialists. This involved Harry's desire to be comfortable and being clear that heroin was what made him feel that way and the staff concerns about potential overdose and 'opiate abuse'. The conversations Harry told me others were having about him, and usually not with him, suggested that concerns about overdose were evident even in palliative care settings. Harry believed that providing opportunities for on demand self-administration of opioids was one way in which these tensions could be resolved.

Regular visits from friends, especially early on when the impact of the liver cancer diagnosis was still being understood, also created difficult conversations with staff about who was allowed to visit and why they were visiting. Staff had concerns about friends providing extra illicit opioids – which they sometimes were. Harry told me people did this as a favour to him and at other times he initiated it because he wanted (or needed) a top up to his dose. The potential role for 'patient peers/advocates' to support staff and Harry was noted especially with the context of a very structured tertiary hospital (Magidson et al., 2021). The demands on staff time without an understanding of harm reduction and on-going drug use meant there could be miscommunication. Recent research (Thandi and Browne, 2019) suggests that abstinence is not a necessary or realistic goal for many older people and there is a specific role for people using drugs themselves as advocates in the palliative care space (Higgs et al., 2020).

Despite Harry being articulate and knowledgeable about both drug use and hepatitis C, he had limited previous exposure to the health care system beyond the emergency department. It was clear that the 'health care system' has not been set up well to work in the best interests of individuals (especially older drug users) with specific needs as they approach end of life. Support is required to help navigate a way through the system and this is where the patient/peer advocate role could be so important (Östlund et al., 2019). Observing the process of having to move around different hospital wards (often without much notice) and then on to palliative care required becoming familiar with the different ways in which hospital wards are run. The process of negotiating and understanding who is 'in charge', how best to 'make friends with' key staff and what, if any, specific rules existed all needed to be worked through. This is as much an issue in the tertiary hospital setting as it is when working with community and residential care settings.

Seemingly simple day-to-day tasks that could be managed individually prior to care, including smoking of cigarettes and daily dosing of pharmacotherapy are complicated by the running of the hospital wards. Not having a suitable smoking space close by the hospital bed and limited availability of staff to support the trip in a wheelchair to the 'smoking areas' meant extra stress for all concerned. The inconsistent timing and delivery of prescribed drugs (including opiate agonist therapy) made for on-going potentially uncomfortable conversations. In Harry's case, he would ask tersely 'Why was my dose so late today'? putting staff on the defensive.

The management of the use of illicit opioids on the ward is extremely challenging for staff and families. Concerns raised by health care staff (professionally trained and not) about the use of opioids at later stages of life for people who have long histories of using opioids show that drug use (especially injecting drugs use) is not well understood. These attitudes appear to come with many of the socialised and stigmatised attitudes to drug use outside of medical settings that have been documented in the literature (Chan Carusone et al., 2019; Strike et al., 2020). The lack of explicit policies for managing the issue was challenging for staff and for families and only meant that patients themselves did what they could to avoid people knowing about their use.

While there is greater awareness in the palliative care sector of the older person using illicit drugs, this normally comes from the experience of working with people who are on opiate agonist therapy (McPherson et al., 2019). There is clearly much less awareness in the aged care space. Partly this reflects the lower health literacy levels of staff in these settings, but this also highlights the need for core skill competencies for staff, both registered health care professionals and unregistered care workers (Palesy and Jakimowicz, 2020; Poulos et al., 2021). Education is also required especially in specific aspects of working with the older person using drugs. This includes education for those working in the in-patient residential settings about the use of naloxone in settings where opioids have been prescribed, including the use of methadone in hospice settings (McPherson et al., 2019).

Finally, it is worth reminding ourselves that, as noted by the main body representing people who use drugs in Australia, AIVL, that this is currently a hidden population (AIVL, 2019). Any work we can do to build awareness and capacity of both the professional and non-professional health care staff in the aged and palliative care sectors to respond positively to the needs of this population will be appreciated by people using drugs and their families and provide an improved quality of care at end of life.

References

Adams, R.J., Howard, N., Tucker, G., Appleton, S., Taylor, A.W., Chittleborough, C., Gill, T., Ruffin, R.E. and Wilson, D.H. (2009) 'Effects of area deprivation on health risks and outcomes: a multilevel, cross-sectional, Australian population study.' *International Journal of Public Health*, 54, pp. 183–192. DOI: 10.1007/s00038-009-7113-x

Anderson, T.L. and Levy, J.A. (2003) 'Marginality among older injectors in today's illicit drug culture: assessing the impact of ageing.' *Addiction*, 98, pp. 761–770. DOI: 10.1046/j.1360-0443.2003.00388.x

Australian Hepatitis Council. (2003) *A sense of belonging, national hepatitis C needs assessment*. Canberra: Australian Government Department of Health and Ageing.

Australian Injecting and Illicit Drug Users League (AIVL). (2019) *A hidden population: supporting healthy ageing for people who inject drugs and/or receive pharmacotherapies*. Canberra: AIVL.

Australian Institute of Health and Welfare (2021). *National Opioid Pharmacotherapy Statistics Annual Data collection*. Cat. no. PHE 266. Canberra: AIHW. Online access: https://www.aihw.gov.au/reports/alcohol-other-drug-treatment-services/national-opioidpharmacotherapy-statistics

Australian Institute of Health and Welfare (AIHW). (2020) *National opioid pharmacotherapy statistics annual data (NOPSAD) collection 2019*. Canberra: Australian Institute of Health and Welfare.

Beynon, C., Mcveigh, J. and Roe, B. (2007) 'Problematic drug use, ageing and older people: trends in the age of drug users in northwest England.' *Ageing and Society*, 27, pp. 799–810. DOI: 10.1017/S0144686X07006411

Beynon, C., Roe, B., Duffy, P. and Pickering, L. (2009) 'Self reported health status, and health service contact, of illicit drug users aged 50 and over: a qualitative interview study in Merseyside, United Kingdom.' *BMC Geriatrics*, 9, p. 45. DOI: 10.1186/1471-2318-9-45

Beynon, C., Stimson, G. and Lawson, E. (2010) 'Illegal drug use in the age of ageing.' *British Journal of General Practice*, 60, pp. 481–482. DOI: 10.3399/bjgp10X514710

Blow, F. (1998) Substance abuse among older adults. *In:* SAMSHA (ed.) *Center for Substance Abuse Treatment*. DHHS publication no. (sma) 98–3179. Rockville, MD.

Bluthenthal, R.N., Simpson, K., Ceasar, R.C., Zhao, J., Wenger, L. and Kral, A.H. (2020) 'Opioid withdrawal symptoms, frequency, and pain characteristics as correlates of health risk among people who inject drugs.' *Drug and Alcohol Dependence*, 211, p. 107932. DOI: 10.1016/j.drugalcdep.2020.107932

Chan Carusone, S., Guta, A., Robinson, S., Tan, D.H., Cooper, C., O'Leary, B., de Prinse, K., Cobb, G., Upshur, R. and Strike, C. (2019) '"Maybe if i stop the drugs, then maybe they'd care?"—hospital care experiences of people who use drugs.' *Harm Reduction Journal*, 16, p. 16. DOI: 10.1186/s12954-019-0285-7

Chang, K-C., Lin, C-Y., Chang, C-C., Ting, S-Y., Cheng, C-M. and Wang, J-D. (2019) 'Psychological distress mediated the effects of self-stigma on quality of life in opioid-dependent individuals: a cross-sectional study.' *PLoS One*, 14, p. e0211033. DOI: 10.1371/journal.pone.0211033

Clarke, J.G., Stein, M.D., McGarry, K.A. and Gogineni, A. (2001) 'Interest in smoking cessation among injection drug users.' *American Journal of Addiction*, 10, pp. 159–166. DOI: 10.1080/105504901750227804

Coupland, H., Day, C., Levy, M.T. and Maher, L. (2009) 'Promoting equitable access to hepatitis C treatment for Indo-chinese injecting drug users.' *Health Promotion Journal of Australia*, 20, pp. 234–240. DOI: 10.1071/HE09234

Crofts, N. and Aitken, C.K. (1997) 'Incidence of bloodborne virus infection and risk behaviours in a cohort of injecting drug users in Victoria, 1990–1995.' *Medical Journal of Australia*, 167, pp. 17–20. DOI: 10.5694/j.1326-5377.1997.tb138757.x.

Dietze, P., Jolley, D., Fry, C. and Bammer, G. (2005) 'Transient changes in behaviour lead to heroin overdose: results from a case-crossover study of non-fatal overdose.' *Addiction*, 100, pp. 636–642. DOI: 10.1111/j.1360-0443.2005.01051.x

Dwyer, R., Topp, L., Maher, L., Power, R., Hellard, M., Walsh, N., Jauncey, M., Conroy, A., Lewis, J. and Aitken, C.K. (2009) 'Prevalences and correlates of non-viral injecting-related injuries and diseases in a convenience sample of Australian injecting drug users.' *Drug and Alcohol Dependence*, 100, pp. 9–16. DOI: 10.1016/j.drugalcdep.2008.08.016

Gossop, M. and Moos, R. (2008) 'Substance misuse among older adults: a neglected but treatable problem.' *Addiction*, 103, pp. 347–348. DOI: 10.1111/j.1360-0443.2007.02096.x.

Goutzamanis, S., Doyle, J.S., Thompson, A., Dietze, P., Hellard, M., Higgs, P. and on behalf of the TAP study group. (2018) 'Experiences of liver health related uncertainty and self-reported stress among people who inject drugs living with hepatitis C virus: a qualitative study.' *BMC Infectious Diseases*, 18, p. 151. DOI: 10.1186/s12879-018-3057-1

Hagan, H., des Jarlais, D., Stern, R., Lelutiu-Weinberger, C., Scheinmann, R., Strauss, S. and Flom, P.L. (2007) 'HCV synthesis project: preliminary analyses of HCV prevalence in relation to age and duration of injection.' *International Journal of Drug Policy*, 18, pp. 341–351. DOI: 10.1016/j.drugpo.2007.01.016

Han, B.H., Cotton, B.P., Polydorou, S., Sherman, S., Ferris, R., Arcila-Mesa, M., Qian, Y. and McNeely, J. (2022) 'Geriatric conditions among middle-aged and older adults on methadone maintenance treatment: a pilot study.' *Journal of Addiction Medicine*, 16, 1, pp. 110–113. DOI: 10.1097/ADM.0000000000000808

Heard, S., Iversen, J., Geddes, L. and Maher, L. (2020) *Australian NSP survey: prevalence of HIV, HCV and injecting and sexual behaviour among NSP attendees, 25-year national data report 1995–2019.* Sydney: The Kirby Institute, UNSW.

Higgs, P. (2015) 'Primary health care and other social issues for older people who inject drugs.' *Drug and Alcohol Research Connection*, 7. Online access at: http://www.connections.edu. au/opinion/primary-health-care-and-other-social-issues-older-people-who-inject-drugs#

Higgs, P., Byrne, J., Yarwood, G., Rumbold, B., Wright, S., Witham, G. and Galvani, S. (2020) 'Highlighting the palliative care needs of people using drugs.' *Collegian*, 27, pp. 581–582. DOI: 10.1016/j.colegn.2020.02.006

Higgs, P. and Dietze, P. (2017) 'Injecting drug use continues in older drug users too.' *British Medical Journal*, 359, p. j4738. DOI: 10.1136/bmj.j4738

Higgs, P., Dwyer, R., Duong, D., Thach, M-L., Hellard, M., Power, R. and Maher, L. (2009) 'Heroin-gel capsule cocktails and groin injecting practices among ethnic Vietnamese in Melbourne, Australia.' *International Journal of Drug Policy*, 20, pp. 340–346. DOI: 10.1016/j.drugpo.2008.05.001

Ho, H. and Maher, L. (2008) 'Có vay có tra (What goes around comes around): culture, risk and vulnerability to blood-borne viral infection among ethnic Vietnamese IDUs.' *Drug Alcohol Review*, 27, pp. 420–428. DOI: 10.1080/09595230801914743

Hser, Y.L, Huang, D., Chou, C. P. and Anglin, M.D. (2007) 'Trajectories of heroin addiction: growth mixture modeling results based on a 33-year follow-up study.' *Evaluation Review*, 31, pp. 548–563. DOI: 10.1177/0193841X07307315

Laslett, A-M., Dietze, P. and Dwyer, R. (2008) 'The oral health of street-recruited injecting drug users: prevalence and correlates of problems.' *Addiction*, 103, pp. 1821–1825. DOI: 10.1111/j.1360-0443.2008.02339.x

Madden, A. and Parkes, P. (2010) 'Coming of age - issues for older opiod injectors.' *Drug and Alcohol Review*, 29(Suppl), p. 47.

Magidson, J.F., Regan, S., Powell, E., Jack, H.E., Herman, G.E., Zaro, C., Kane, M.T. and Wakeman, S.E. (2021) 'Peer recovery coaches in general medical settings: changes in utilization, treatment engagement, and opioid use.' *Journal of Substance Abuse Treatment*, 122, p. 108248. DOI: 10.1016/j.jsat.2020.108248

Maher, L., Jalaludin, B., Chant, K. Jayasuriya, R., Sladden, T., Kkaldor, J.M. and Sargent, P.L. (2006) 'Incidence and risk factors for hepatitis c seroconversion in injecting drug users in Australia.' *Addiction*, 101, pp. 1499–1508. DOI: 10.1111/j.1360-0443.2006.01543.x

Mateu-Gelabert, P., Sandoval, M., Meylakhs, P., Wendel, T. and Friedman, S.R. (2010) 'Strategies to avoid opiate withdrawal: implications for HCV and HIV risks.' *International Journal of Drug Policy*, 21, pp. 179–185. DOI: 10.1016/j.drugpo.2009.08.007

Mattick, R.P., Kimber, J., Breen, C. and Davoli, M. (2008) 'Buprenorphine maintenance versus placebo or methadone maintenance for opioid dependence.' *Cochrane Database Syst Review*, cd002207. DOI: 10.1002/14651858.CD002207.pub3

Mayock, P. and Butler, S. (2021) '"I'm always hiding and ducking and diving": the stigma of growing older on methadone.' *Drugs: Education, Prevention and Policy*, pp. 1–11. DOI: 10.1080/09687637.2021.1886253

McCoy, C.B., Metsch, L.R., Chitwood, D. and Miles, C. (2001) 'Drug use and barriers to use of health care services.' *Substance Use and Misuse*, 36, pp. 789–806. DOI: 10.1081/JA-100104091

McPherson, M.L., Walker, K.A., Davis, M.P., Bruera, E., Reddy, A., Paice, J., Malotte, K., Lockman, D.K., Wellman, C., sSlpeter, S., Bemben, N.M., Ray, J.B., Lapointe, B.J. and Chou, R. (2019) 'Safe and appropriate use of methadone in hospice and palliative care: expert consensus white paper.' *Journal of Pain and Symptom Management*, 57, pp. 635–645.e4. DOI: 10.1016/j.jpainsymman.2018.12.001

Morgan, N., Daniels, W. and Subramaney, U. (2020) 'An inverse relationship between alcohol and heroin use in heroin users post detoxification.' *Substance Abuse and Rehabilitation*, 11, pp. 1–8. DOI: 10.2147/SAR.S228224

Morgan, K., Lee, J. and Sebar, B. (2015) 'Community health workers: a bridge to healthcare for people who inject drugs.' *International Journal of Drug Policy*, 26, pp. 380–387. DOI: 10.1016/j.drugpo.2014.11.001

Murphy, N., Karlin-Zysman, C. and Anandan, S. (2018) 'Management of chronic pain in the elderly: a review of current and upcoming novel therapeutics.' *American Journal of Therapeutics*, 25, 1, p. e36. DOI: 10.1097/MJT.0000000000000659

Niederau, C., Lange, S., Heintges, T., Erhardt, A., Buschkamp, M., Hurter, D., Nawrocki, M., Kruska, L., Hensel, F., Petry, W. and Haussinger, D. (1998) 'Prognosis of chronic hepatitis C: results of a large, prospective cohort study.' *Hepatology*, 28, pp. 1687–1695. DOI: 10.1002/hep.510280632

Oppenheimer, E., Tobutt, C., Taylor, C. and Andrew, T. (1994) Death and survival in a cohort of heroin addicts from london clinics: a 22-year follow-up study. *Addiction*, 89, pp. 1299–1308. DOI: 10.1111/j.1360-0443.1994.tb03309.x

Östlund, U., Blomberg, K., Söderman, A. and Werkander Harstäde, C. (2019) 'How to conserve dignity in palliative care: suggestions from older patients, significant others, and healthcare professionals in Swedish municipal care.' *BMC Palliative Care*, 18, p. 10. DOI: 10.1186/s12904-019-0393-x

Palesy, D. and Jakimowicz, S. (2020) 'Health literacy support for Australian home-based care recipients: a role for homecare workers?' *Home Health Care Services Quarterly*, 39, pp. 17–32. DOI: 10.1080/01621424.2019.1691698

Parkes, P. (2010) *Double jeopardy: a discussion paper on the existence and needs of a cohort of older injecting opioid users in Australia.* Canberra: AIVL.

Pawlotsky, J-M., Feld, J., Zeuzem, S. and Hoofnagle, J.H. (2015) 'From non-A, non-B hepatitis to hepatitis C virus cure.' *Journal of Hepatology*, 62, pp. s87–s99. DOI: 10.1016/j.jhep.2015.02.006

Poulos, R.G., Boon, M.Y., George, A., Liu, K.P.Y., Mak, M., Maurice, C., Palesy, D., Pont, L.G., Poulos, C.J., Ramsey, S., Simpson, P., Steiner, G.Z., Villarosa, A.R., Watson, K. and Parker, D. (2021) 'Preparing for an aging Australia: the development of multidisciplinary core competencies for the Australian health and aged care workforce.' *Gerontology and Geriatrics Education*, 42, pp. 399–422. DOI: 10.1080/02701960.2020.1843454

Radcliffe, P. and Stevens, A. (2008) 'Are drug treatment services only for 'thieving junkie scumbags'? Drug users and the management of stigmatised identities.' *Social Science and Medicine*, 67, pp. 1065–1073. DOI: 10.1016/j.socscimed.2008.06.004

Richmond, J. (2009) *Do you C what i C? National hepatitis C needs assessment 2008.* Canberra, Australia: Hepatitis Australia.

Rosenburg, H. (1995) 'The elderly and the use of illicit drugs: sociological and epidemiological considerations.' *Substance Use and Misuse*, 30, pp. 1925–1951. DOI: 10.3109/10826089509071061

Rowe, J. (2008) *A raw deal? Impact on the health of consumers relative to the cost of pharmacotherapy.* The Salvation Army, Research and Advocacy Unit; Royal Melbourne Institute of Technology (Australia). Centre for Applied Social Research.

Salter, H., Hutton, J., Cantwell, K., Dietze, P., Higgs, P., Straub, A., Zordan, R. and Lloyd-Jones, M. (2020) 'Review article: Rapid review of the emergency department-initiated buprenorphine for opioid use disorder.' *Emergency Medicine Australasia*, 32, pp. 924–934. DOI: 10.1111/1742-6723.13654

Shepard, C.W., Finelli, L. and Alter, M.J. (2005) 'Global epidemiology of hepatitis C virus infection.' *Lancet Infectious Diseases*, 5, pp. 558–567. DOI: 10.1016/S1473-3099(05)70216-4

Stoové, M.A., Gifford, S.M. and Dore, G.J. (2005) 'The impact of injecting drug use status on hepatitis c related referral and treatment.' *Drug and Alcohol Dependence*, 77, pp. 81–86. DOI: 10.1016/j.drugalcdep.2004.07.002

Strike, C., Robinson, S., Guta, A., Tan, D.H., O'Leary, B., Cooper, C., Upshur, R. and Chan Carusone, S. (2020) 'Illicit drug use while admitted to hospital: patient and health care provider perspectives.' *PLoS One*, 15, p. e0229713. DOI: 10.1371/journal.pone.0229713

Sutherland, R., Uporova, J., Chandrasena, U., Price, O., Karlsson, A., Gibbs, D., Swanton, R., Bruno, R., Dietze, P., Lenton, S., Salom, C. Daly, C., Thomas, N., Juckel, J., Agramunt, S., Wilson, Y., Woods, E., Moon, C., Degenhardt, L., Farrell, M. and Peacock, A. (2021) *Australian drug trends 2021: Key findings from the National Illicit Drug Reporting System (IDRS) INTERVIEWS.* Sydney: National Drug and Alcohol Research Centre, UNSW Sydney.

Thandi, M.K.G. and Browne, A.J. (2019) 'The social context of substance use among older adults: implications for nursing practice.' *Nursing Open*, 6, pp. 1299–1306. DOI: 10.1002/nop2.339

Tobutt, C., Oppenheimer, E. and Laranjeira, R. (1996) 'Health of cohort of heroin addicts from London clinics: 22 year follow up.' *BMJ*, 312, p. 1458. DOI: 10.1136/bmj.312.7044.1458

Tuchman, E. (2003) 'Methadone and menopause: midlife women in drug treatment.' *Journal of Social Work Practice in the Addictions*, 3, pp. 43–55. DOI: 10.1300/J160v03n02_04

Winter, R., Nguyen, O., Higgs, P., Armstrong, S., Duong, D., Thach, M-L., Aitken, C.K. and Hellard, M. (2008) 'Integrating enhanced hepatitis c testing and counselling in research.' *International Journal of Drug Policy*, 19, pp. 66–70. DOI: 10.1016/j.drugpo.2007.04.002

Xiao, L.D., Harrington, A., Mavromaras, K., Ratcliffe, J., Mahuteau, S., Isherwood, L. and Gregoric, C. (2021) 'Care workers' perspectives of factors affecting a sustainable aged care workforce.' *International Nursing Review*, 68, pp. 49–58. DOI: 10.1111/inr.12635

Yarnell, S., Li, L., MacGrory, B., Trevisan, L. and Kirwin, P. (2020) 'Substance use disorders in later life: a review and synthesis of the literature of an emerging public health concern.' *The American Journal of Geriatric Psychiatry*, 28, pp. 226–236. DOI: 10.1016/j.jagp.2019.06.005

Part III

Social inequalities

Introduction by Sam Wright

The chapters in Part III address social inequalities and their interplay with health inequalities, deprivation and marginalisation. This final section of the book repositions our primary focus from health inequalities (relating to differential health literacy, intellectual disabilities, mental health difficulties, ageing and Hepatitis C), to wider considerations of social inequalities. This is not to suggest that health and social factors are discrete issues that can be considered in isolation, but rather to layer up our understanding in a way that appreciates the complex interaction between health and social factors. By introducing a specific focus on social inequalities, we bring in recognition of the structural, gendered, racialised and intersectional aspects of both substance use and access to health and social care.

The four chapters contained in this section examine particular social identities and the structural barriers to accessing health and social care that they pose. In Chapter 9, Brophy and Colclough describe their work with people experiencing homelessness who need end-of-life care and are using substances, challenging common palliative care assumptions that: (1) people have a home in which they can be cared for; (2) they have friends and family around them to provide informal care; (3) they will actively protect their own health and (4) feel sufficient self-worth to access and pursue healthcare. In Chapter 10, Brien tells how she built a trusting relationship with Jane who was terminally ill but continuing in sex work. In this heart-rending account of one woman's end of life, we are intimately drawn into the delicate task of engaging and supporting Jane whose shame of her situation and sense of obligation towards her partner had been preventing her from getting the care that she needed. Chapter 11, written by Ahmed and Chesterton, highlights the challenges and inequalities facing Black and minoritised communities in accessing substance use, palliative and end-of-life services. The authors describe how the layering of deprivation, health inequalities, structural racism and marginalisation results in unmet needs, reduced quality of life and missed opportunities for advance care planning. But more than this, they highlight both the exclusionary nature of the Christian background of many hospices as well as the fact that our very understanding of what a 'good death' is, has been rooted in Western ethics which ignore the important role of different faiths. Peacock and

DOI: 10.4324/9781003187882-11

Turner in Chapter 12 consider substance use, disadvantage and end-of-life care for people in prison. Pointing out that deprivation of liberty is the criminal justice punishment, they highlight that prisoners should receive the same standards of health care available in the community, yet the ageing effects of imprisonment and the paucity of specialist health provision for people in prison often leave prison officers and fellow prisoners the sole providers of social care for those experiencing frailty.

These chapters reveal the shared experiences of marginalised people who use substances and are approaching the end of their life: feeling excluded from health/ social care decision-making, low expectations about professional support, and facing huge access barriers due to social disapproval. We see the direct impact of stigma and discrimination, but also witness the very real impact that the compassion of individual practitioners makes.

9 Homelessness and substance use within palliative and end-of-life care

Niamh Brophy and Alison Colclough

Introduction

Homelessness is a poignant word, one that may conjure up negative images of rough sleepers not from the local community and who have themselves to blame for the situation they find themselves in through poor choices (Leibowitz and Kruger, 2013). These are enduring negative stereotypes that over-simplify a complex issue, and exacerbate exclusion for all those affected by homelessness, whether they fit those stereotypes or not. The routes into homelessness are multiple and complex, and many factors influence the likelihood of someone becoming homeless and the length of time they will remain homeless. What is clear from the decades of research referenced within this chapter is that homelessness is not a static state of being, but a complex and dynamic experience influenced by a range of factors – social, psychological, physical and practical – meaning that no one individual's experience is the same (see Table 9.1). The causes of homelessness and experiences of each individual are very different.

What connect these experiences are multiple layers of inequity, including: poverty, stigma, abuse and exclusion. They often lead these individuals to become invisible to services whose task it is to support them, particularly when substance use is involved. We must understand these issues and how they interact with each other if we are to improve the experiences for people affected by homelessness as they come to the end of their lives.

The duration of homelessness also needs consideration. We acknowledge that, for many people, homelessness can be a short-lived experience, due to a job loss or housing shortage. For the purpose of this chapter, we will be focussing on chronic homelessness; that is, individuals who remain continuously homeless for a year or longer or for those who have a disabling condition and experience four episodes of homelessness over a two-year period (Fazel et al., 2014). Those entrenched in the cycle of homelessness often experience social and health deprivation alongside substance dependence and multiple morbidities. This is the group of people who we have most experience with as practitioners; they have high levels of complex needs that go unmet by mainstream services.

Chronic homelessness is typically characterised by poor physical and mental health, combined with substance use issues (tri-morbidity) (Cornes et al., 2018).

DOI: 10.4324/9781003187882-12

Table 9.1 Types of homelessness explained

Types of homelessness	
Rough sleeping	The most extreme end of the homelessness spectrum. Anyone who is sleeping outside.
Statutory homeless	This includes anyone registered as homeless with their local authority and placed in emergency or temporary accommodation. Types of temporary accommodation: local authority hostels, hotels, bed and breakfast accommodation (B&Bs)
Hidden homeless	This includes sofa surfing, living in squats, hostels
At risk of homelessness	Individuals or households living in insecure (spending more than 50% of their income on rent) or unsuitable accommodation

Adapted from Shelter.org (2021).

Estimates of substance use among people experiencing homelessness in the UK vary. Alcohol dependence estimates range from 8.1 to 58.5% and drug dependence estimates range from 4.5 to 54.2% among homeless populations (Fazel et al., 2008). This tri-morbidity is both a cause and consequence of a complex interplay of factors including childhood trauma, poverty, lack of social support and legacies of abuse which have a significant impact on an individual's health and mental health (Luchenski et al., 2018). These experiences demonstrate Hart's classic inverse care law; those groups most in need of support have the most difficulty accessing care (Hart, 1971). For those experiencing homelessness, this results in high rates of multi-morbidity and early mortality, with deaths occurring much earlier than the housed population (Queen et al., 2017).

Early onset frailty and geriatric conditions are also common among those experiencing homelessness with substance use problems (Rogans-Watson et al., 2020). Yet often these individuals will remain in hostels or other temporary accommodation with little to no input from health and social care services. Treatable medical conditions are common causes of death among this group, as are deaths related to alcohol and drug use (Aldridge et al., 2018). This culminates in mortality rates that are often two to five times higher than even the most deprived housed populations (Aldridge et al., 2018). In the UK, for example, the mean age of death for someone sleeping rough is 46 for males, and 43 for females (ONS, 2020). Little is known about the end-of-life experiences of people who are homeless, with deaths happening suddenly in hostels, on the streets or in hospitals (Thomas, 2012). There is some high-quality quantitative and qualitative research in existence that examines homelessness, palliative and end-of-life care, but this is limited (Witham et al., 2019a). Given the high symptom burden of this group and the prevalence of multiple, long-term health conditions, access to palliative care should be a part of their care planning.

Within this chapter, we have referenced current research that reflects what we are seeing in everyday practice. The research we do have informs us that people experiencing homelessness who are using substances (PEHUS – People Experiencing Homelessness Using Substances will be used from now on) face a number of barriers to care, including a lack of referral to palliative care services, stigma, discrimination and systems which are often rigid and inflexible, with professionals lacking the skills and knowledge to support them.

As this chapter develops, we will look in more depth at some of these gaps, the reasons for them and ways to facilitate better ways of working to overcome them. We acknowledge that palliative and end-of-life care are broad terms that encompass a wide range of important issues. For the purpose of this chapter, we will be using these terms interchangeably and discussing palliative care as it applies to the management and support of individuals with complex needs and non-curable illnesses who are deemed to be in the last year of life. We hope to contribute to the learning and confidence of practitioners working in the field of health and social care in order to better prepare them to deliver high standard palliative and end-of-life care to some of the most complex and vulnerable members of our society; ensuring that people who are homeless and use substances can live well and die in a place of their choosing.

Homelessness, palliative care and substance use: challenges in accessing support

Individual and interpersonal challenges

We must first understand something of the lived experience of PEHUS in order to know how best to care and support them as they come to the end of their lives. We will use the following case study to draw out the key individual challenges in accessing palliative care experienced by PEHUS.

Learning points

Trauma

Sharon had experienced such relational trauma throughout her life that she had no trust in staff or professionals. Consequently, no one felt they really knew her, or were best placed to support her to live well and have those difficult conversations about her end-of-life choices.

Maguire et al.'s (2009) systematic review found that traumatic experiences strongly predict homelessness later in life. The *Hard Edges* report found that 85% of people who are homeless, sex working or in touch with criminal justice services experienced trauma, with these events often occurring in childhood (Bramley and Fitzpatrick, 2015). These traumatic experiences or ACES (Adverse Childhood Experiences) can be psychological/physical/sexual in nature. They lay the foundations for a world view that people cannot be trusted, that the world is unsafe and that emotions are so painful they need to be numbed.

Case study: Sharon

Sharon had been intermittently homeless all of her adult life. She was placed in the care of the local authority at the age of 12, following physical and sexual abuse by family members since the age of 6. Foster homes struggled to manage Sharon's behaviour and she moved homes often throughout her adolescence. When she turned 18 she found she did not have the life skills to live independently, manage a tenancy or get a job. She quickly became homeless, relying on sex work for income. Without a role model or someone to teach her how to understand and express her emotions in a healthy way, she turned to drugs and found them to be an effective tool for numbing her feelings. By the age of 37, Sharon was a long-term heavy drinker and injecting drug user. She had multiple complex health problems as a result of her substance use, including liver disease and HIV, as well as a history of numerous suicide attempts and episodes of self-harm. She engaged sporadically with staff at the hostel she was living in, as well as with mental health and substance use services, but would quickly be discharged due to non-engagement. Following one crisis admission to A&E she was told by doctors she would not live longer than a year if she continued to be non-compliant with her medication and use substances. Sharon expressed she did not intend to reduce her substance use: she found the world too overwhelming if she did not have access to drugs. Because of this, her options for care and support were limited given that most services operated a zero tolerance policy around alcohol and drug use. As a result, Sharon remained in a hostel as her health deteriorated. Hostel staff became anxious that Sharon would die soon – not least because they had no medical or nurse training and did not provide personal care. Sharon remained in her accommodation with limited support and died in hospital six hours after admission.

The experience of homelessness itself can also be traumatic, as it certainly was for Sharon. This trauma can be due to the increased exposure to violence or assault, or from not having a home and all that goes with it: social support, connection, a place of physical safety. Previous exposure to trauma and the presence of corresponding symptoms are correlated with an increase in reported pain and distress in clinical patients (Otis et al., 2003). However, service staff can also re-trigger trauma in someone who has been traumatised if they do not take a trauma-informed approach to care. The principles of this approach focus on education, safety and empowerment to create the conditions needed to heal from traumatic events and build healthy relational connections with others.

For Sharon, palliative intervention was preceded by years of trauma, abuse, deteriorating health and medical emergencies. These experiences are of concern to any palliative care professional as they impact on a person's engagement and utilisation of the service.

Dual diagnosis

Sharon had a 'dual diagnosis' consisting of substance use dependence and mental illness. This combination of diagnoses can reveal a disconnect between specialist mental health and substance use services and the individual themselves due to the demands placed upon them by services (PHE, 2017). They face practical and organisational barriers such as inflexible appointment times or attendance policies, increasing the risk that they may 'fall through the gap' between services when no single professional team takes the lead (Shulman et al., 2018). A number of times Sharon was discharged from mental health services because of her substance use, yet substance use services felt her mental health was the priority need, which meant she was unable to access either form of support. This is not an uncommon experience.

It is essential to take a multi-disciplinary team planning (MDT) approach in these complex cases: early intervention and MDT planning are crucial. Involving all professionals in that person's care will ensure the individual remains at the centre of discussions is supported holistically, and given the best quality of care possible. Practical considerations like pain management plans can be considered alongside individual wishes and needs for future care.

Competing priorities

Sharon, like many PEHUS, struggled to attend appointments for her physical or mental health. This is a common barrier for PEHUS accessing any kind of health care (Purkey and MacKenzie, 2019). When basic needs have not been met like food, shelter, clothing; healthcare can shift lower down on the list of priorities. Individuals must have the capacity to prioritise their health over other concerns but if substance dependence needs to be managed, this may be unlikely to happen.

Interpersonal challenges and implications for practitioners – trust, stigma and shame

Previous negative experiences of health or social care settings can lead to PEHUS avoiding care altogether to avoid feeling shame and being stigmatised (Purkey and MacKenzie, 2019). These feelings can be so great as to supersede the perceived need for medical intervention.

As palliative care professionals, we are mindful of our interactions with PEHUS given the likelihood that they may struggle to have trust in us. Table 9.2 gives some pointers as to how to improve outcomes with PEHUS. Trust is essential to develop a therapeutic alliance with a patient, and for adequate pain management. Both of these factors are crucial to be able to provide good quality palliative care. Prescribers must explore the patient's experience and reporting of pain levels and trust their account to prescribe adequate levels of pain relief (Witham et al., 2019b). Without these honest conversations taking place, particularly when substance use is involved, pain may not be managed adequately and could serve to exacerbate the feelings of mistrust between patient and health professional.

Table 9.2 Top tips and recommendations

Top tips and recommendations for improving outcomes when working with PEHUS

- Build trust and a therapeutic alliance by taking a trauma-informed approach to your practice
- Consider peer advocacy
- Person-centred care, placing the individual at the centre of all discussions and where appropriate involving them in all aspects of decision making
- Collaborative MDT working involving all those who are engaged in and supporting the individual, e.g. health, housing, mental health, substance use, social care, advocacy services.

Individual and service development top tips

- Consider creating a *homeless/palliative care champion* within each service team
- Utilise *peer advocates* and people with lived experience in planning and delivery of services
- Design services with the needs of PEHUS in mind: be *flexible, realistic*, non-punitive; keep the person at the centre of all plans
- Respond to local need and encourage *open access* and *in reach* models of care
- Be *accepting of uncertainty* in relation to illness trajectories
- Be *informed* about trauma, addiction, mental health and harm reduction approaches to care
- Work in an *integrated, multi-disciplinary* way encouraging sharing of information and shared care practices
- *Have cultural sensitivity* to the needs of PEHUS

Additional challenges: difficulty in recognising dying

The case study below highlights some of the difficulties in recognising dying for PEHUS. Living in a hostel, being relatively young, not having close relationships with individuals who can advocate for the person, combined with illnesses such as liver failure and still using substances means that recognising dying is not simple (Shulman et al., 2017).

Recognising deteriorating health and dying

Research suggests that 50% of people with decompensated liver failure will die within two years and those who continue to drink, much sooner (Dolan and Arnold, 2015). Mark had been told by the hepatology team that he would likely die in the next 12 months if he carried on drinking, but they did not refer him to local palliative care services. Late referral to palliative care for PEHUS remains a major barrier to care, as does people's reticence to access palliative care, feeling that: 'it's not for people like me' (Klop et al., 2018, McNeil, 2012, 2013). It was the hostel team who recognised Mark's deteriorating health and the possibility he could be dying. They knew him well and witnessed the increasingly frequent hospital admissions and general deterioration in everyday life. They informed the

> **Case study: Mark – Part 1**
>
> *Mark was 37 and living in a hostel. He had been drinking since his teens and his family said he had been a 'wild child', never able to concentrate or settle to anything and always in trouble. He had decompensated liver disease that necessitated stays in hospital at least once a month to have his abdomen drained. Mark consistently forgot to take his medications, could not walk far enough to reach the local corner shop and some days struggled to manage the stairs in the hostel. He was sleeping for long periods of time and eating only small amounts. Although young in years, his body was that of a much older person, as is not uncommon in PEHUS (Rogans-Watson et al., 2020). Poor nutrition, competing priorities including substance use, physical and mental health problems, all contributed to Mark ageing much more rapidly than the general population.*

local hospice palliative care coordinator (PCC) as she had delivered training in the hostel around palliative and end-of-life care, and this led to the local hospice supporting Mark and the homelessness workers.

Learning points

Role of hospices

In the UK, hospices are seen as experts in delivering palliative and end-of-life care. However, many people including social and health care professionals have a misconception that hospices are there simply for end-of-life care (Cagle et al., 2016). A systematic review of inequalities in hospice care by Tobin et al. (2021: 1) concluded that: '*Barriers of prognostic uncertainty, institutional cultures, particular needs of certain groups and lack of public awareness of hospice services remain substantial challenges to the hospice movement in ensuring equitable access for all*'. Hospices still need to open their doors wider to marginalised groups, including PEHUS. Some have started to do this and these tend to have homelessness palliative care coordinators (PCC) who perform various roles, such as educating and training within hostels, advocating for PEHUS and forming strong therapeutic relationships with them. They also work closely across all sectors to include health, social care and homelessness support networks, coordinating these services so the PEHUS are kept at the very centre of care and do not slip through the various gaps in established services (Hospice UK, 2018).

Practitioners need time to build up respectful and trusting relationships. Connecting with someone in the palliative phase rather than the dying phase allows more opportunity for this to happen, as advocated by Klop et al. (2018). They recommend a low threshold, harm minimisation approach, and this is what the hospice practised. Mark was allowed to drink in the hospice and was treated with dignity and respect. Care was tailored to his needs, and he felt secure enough to

---

Case study: Mark – Part 2

The hostel Mark lived in had previously received training from their local hospice which had a homelessness palliative care service. Part of their training was learning about the 'Surprise question': 'Would you be surprised if this person were to die in the next 12 months?' This had become a useful question at the hostel, especially for practitioners who may not have any medical training. It gave them 'permission' to work with the individual. Without this permission, the person had little chance of accessing palliative services. The PCC advocated for Mark and coordinated much of his care through a very complex health and social care system (O'Neil et al., 2012). Mark and the PCC began to work together and a therapeutic relationship was established. Through this relationship he allowed others into his life, such as a Macmillan nurse who managed his symptoms. He won continued health care funding and was accepting of carers. He agreed to go to the hospice for a short stay and eventually the hospice became his preferred place of care and he had a peaceful death there.

---

remain there until he died. Due to the hospice's involvement, his parents were supported during his life and after his death, which is not always the case where substance use is involved (Galvani, 2018).

System challenges

Many of the social and health care systems in the UK are not developed to support this complex group of individuals (Galvani et al., 2019; Galvani and Wright, 2019). For example, within the UK everyone has the right to register with a General Practitioner (GP) in primary care. Without identification, historically PEHUS have been turned away from GP practices despite this being against NHS guidelines which state that a person has the right to access primary care without identification.

Working together for safe prescribing

One of the important principles of good palliative care is symptom management, and that includes pain. Opioids are very commonly used to manage pain, especially cancer pain. Individuals using drugs or alcohol are at risk of being under medicated and left in acute pain (McCreaddie et al., 2010). Some professionals mistakenly feel that the person is asking for analgesia for the 'high' (Bell et al., 2013). Others are scared to prescribe, fearing that it may tip the individual into addiction again. Some do not have the confidence to prescribe to this group especially if there is a methadone prescription in place. Sometimes patients who have had a drug addiction in the past are themselves scared to take opioids, fearing they will trigger old traumas related to their historic drug use, also that if they need to stop taking these opioids then past traumas of withdrawal will be revisited. Prater et al. (2002) argue for the aggressive treatment of pain at end of life and the best way to achieve this is through therapeutic relationships with professionals.

Inflexibility of services

A further challenge is that many services are inflexible (Hudson et al., 2016). Inevitably, appointments are made to suit the needs of the service, not the individual. Missed appointments do not always get followed up, for example, memory problems and cognitive impairment are not uncommon in people drinking excessively and diagnostic overshadowing may lead practitioners to neglect dementia or mental health as a possible cause (RCPsych, 2018).

Hostels

While homeless hostels are more flexible than other forms of accommodation, they are primarily set up for tenancy support. Workers in hostels are not carers and hostels are not registered to give care. Someone with deteriorating health who is living in a hostel or a shared house may need support with medications, food preparation and personal hygiene. Hostels are not made for this high level of need. Ground floor access to showers, rooms that can accommodate a hospital bed and difficulty in getting carers into the hostels at the appropriate times of day, all add to the difficulties of getting adequate care to this group. Table 9.3 highlights these key challenges relating to substance use within the context of homelessness.

Overcoming the challenges: the value of a person-centred approach

We advocate for care to be guided by five broad principles as outlined below:

1   Value-driven, personalised care

We have a collective responsibility to deliver equitable, inclusive care for everyone approaching the end of life. But what does that look like when people and situations are so varied, and circumstances so complex as in the lives of PEHUS? Since individuals are not homogenous, any approach must be guided by broad principles that maximise value and quality for patients – care based on needs and preferences, provided in a way that feels safe and accessible. These broad principles are:

    i   Care is personalised
        For PEHUS this could be offering services such as in-reach nurse support to a hostel, or planning end-of-life care in a hostel setting because that is the place the patient considers their home.

Table 9.3 Key sector challenges in providing palliative care for PEHUS

Drug and alcohol services
- Operate in a recovery focussed landscape; end-of-life care does not fit their philosophy.
- Lack of alcohol-free accommodation ('dry' facilities) to provide people with choice at end of life.
- Difficulty accessing funding for detox/rehab for people approaching the end of life/ who are medically unstable.

Homeless sector & accommodation providers
- Operate in a recovery focussed landscape; end-of-life care does not fit in easily to this philosophy.
- Hostels and temporary accommodation are not designed to be places of care/death (for health and safety and other practical reasons).
- Homeless sector staff do not have medical or nursing backgrounds.
- Hostels and temporary accommodation are not registered to store or administer drugs.
- They do not often provide 24 hour support.

Health and social care
- Difficulty recognising PEHUS as approaching end of life due to:
  - Young age
  - Nature of illnesses
  - Multi morbidity
  - Social determinants of individual conditions.
- Illnesses sometimes seen as 'behavioural' rather than 'end of life'.
- Limited training and awareness of health issues related to multiple deprivation.
- Difficulty determining level of need when an inpatient in hospital and discharge planning (i.e. level of need is not apparent when someone is detoxed from substances, being fed and cared for in clinical environment). Deterioration is common once discharged and support removed.

ii Care is coordinated

With many different services involved, having a named coordinator or service that leads on case management is particularly important as people's wishes and priorities may change quickly as their health deteriorates.

iii Care is provided in a way that assures dignity, compassion and respect.

For a person to receive care that is dignified, compassionate and respectful, we must provide choice and honour the wishes of the people we are working with, even if that goes against our own values and wishes. Table 9.4 explores some questions to consider when supporting PEHUS. Some of us may not think it is dignified to be cared for and die on the streets. We must remember that we are coming with a different set of experiences, values and beliefs that influence our world view and judgement of what is dignified and safe. When someone has capacity and is given choice, their informed decisions must be respected and carried out with compassion wherever possible. We must also have an understanding and sensitivity to patients' feelings of shame and stigma and how it affects their decision-making process.

Table 9.4 Questions to consider when supporting PEHUS

Questions	Considerations
What past events may be influencing how this person is with me right now?	• Previous traumatic experiences • Negative experiences with health and care professionals • Fear of being shamed or stigmatised • Lack of dignity and respect
How can I maximise a sense of trust, safety and respect in my interactions with this person?	• Improve understanding of trauma-informed care • Incorporate the use of strengths-based approaches; highlight resilience and the individual's ability to make their own choices
What competing priorities might make it challenging for them to access support? Can I mitigate these somehow?	• Support to ensure basic needs are met (i.e. food, accommodation, psychological support) • Ensuring adequate opioid/alcohol management plan in place (particularly before admission to hospital as this is a common reason for self-discharge)

2   A shift in focus to work with uncertainty and enable future planning

Given many PEHUS do not get access to palliative care until the last days or weeks of life (Fitzpatrick et al., 2012). We advocate for a shift in focus from end-of-life care to supporting people with advanced ill health. Poor access and engagement with healthcare, coupled with the difficulty in predicting prognoses for people with multiple morbidities or substance use related illnesses (e.g. alcohol related liver disease), means we cannot rely on traditional referral pathways to identify and engage with individuals in their last year of life. Rather, we must be more accepting and flexible in the face of uncertainty with the 'trigger for action' being when an individual's health is *a cause for concern*, for themselves or those who know them.

This shift in focus would enable advanced care planning discussions to happen and people's end-of-life wishes to be identified earlier, so care is not crisis led. Fostering a 'parallel planning approach' – hoping for the best, planning for the worst – would allow professionals to explore an individual's insight into their illness and what their preferences for care might be. This parallel planning approach is highlighted in Figure 9.1. In this approach the professionals are also keeping options open and crucially, not removing hope for an already vulnerable person. This is very important, particularly for people whose illnesses are related to their substance use; it enables them to feel a sense of control and choice over their future, no matter how limited that may be. It also gives professionals a framework to work with uncertainty, given the challenges that present when working with unpredictable prognoses and illness trajectories.

Parallel planning: Exploration of insight and wishes while keeping options open

Hoping for the best
- Exploration of detox and rehab if individual hopes to reduce their substance use
- Goal setting with a manageable and achievable focus

Planning for the worst
- Exploring insight and wishes if substance use does not decrease
- Care planning in the event an acute deterioration occurs again

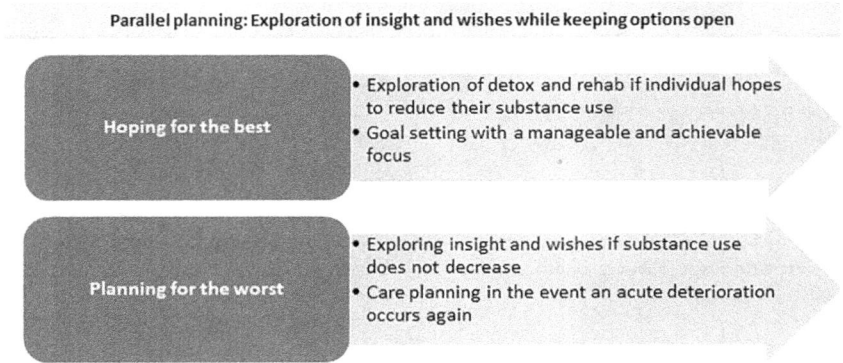

Figure 9.1 A parallel planning approach for a hostel resident with alcohol-related liver disease.

3   Effective communication

Effective communication is essential for delivery of good quality, person-centred care. This means engaging with PEHUS in a way that conveys trust and respect for them as human beings and for their choices, even if, as a professional, you perceive them to be unwise or you hope for something different for them. Gaining an understanding of someone's insight into their illness should be the foundation all future care plans are built upon. For example, you may plan to support someone with end stage liver disease in a very different way if they do not believe anything is wrong with them ('I'm not yellow yet, I'm not as bad as they say!'), versus someone who accepts and understands they are likely to die in the next three to six months.

For this client group the following tool highlighted in Table 9.5 can be used as a prompt to support and facilitate person-centred conversations to identify insight and clarify wishes and priorities for future care.

4   Education, training and collaboration

Given many PEHUS will remain in hostels as they approach the end of their lives (Webb et al., 2018) and will have little access to health and social care support, this places staff in these accommodations in very stressful and difficult situations (Shulman et al., 2017). Exploring different models of person-centred care could improve patient outcomes and support homeless sector staff in these contexts.

It has also been found that providing training and support to hostel staff in matters relating to palliative care can improve their knowledge and confidence in supporting deteriorating health in a hostel setting (Shulman et al., 2018). Upskilling in this way enables earlier identification of people in the last year of life and increases the wellbeing of homeless sector staff by improving their knowledge of palliative care services and how to utilise them appropriately.

Table 9.5 Questions to consider tool

Questions to consider	

Physical health
- What do you understand about your current health condition?
- Have you had any thoughts about where things are going with your illness?
- What are your main concerns at the moment?
- What would you like to see happen next?

Substance Use
- Have you had any thoughts about reducing your drinking/substance use?
- Say you struggled to stop drinking/using, what do you think might happen in the next 3/6/9 months?
- What might the benefits of detox/rehab be right now?
- Can we make a plan to meet again in another week/month, to see where you are at with everything then?

Emotional
- How are you feeling about your recent hospital admission/diagnosis/poor health?
- I've noticed you seem a bit withdrawn lately, can I help with anything?
- What are your main concerns/worries right now?
- What do you feel could help?

Hopes for the future
- What is most important to you right now?
- What does living well mean to you – what would that look like for you right now?
- Are there things you have always wanted to do?
- Would you like support to reconnect with family?

Treatment and care
- If you became very ill, where would you want to be cared for?
- Do you feel you are having any extra difficulty getting around or taking care of yourself lately?
- Would you like to talk to your GP about what treatments options are available to you?

Relationships
- Who are the people you trust the most?
- Who would you like to be there if you were to become ill?
- Who would you not want to be there if you were to become ill?
- Would you like support to reconnect with family?

Social/Practical issues
- Do you have any difficulties attending appointments lately? Could we help with this?
- Have you thought about making a will or a Letter of Wishes? Have you had any thoughts about how you would like to be remembered?

Source: homelesspalliativecare.com

Health and social care professionals may also lack the confidence and skills to work effectively with PEHUS. Adequate training for all sectors working with PEHUS will empower services to engage individuals in ways that are appropriate, accessible and person-centred.

5   Multi-disciplinary team working

Given the complexities in planning end-of-life care for PEHUS, any approach needs to be collaborative and utilise the knowledge and expertise of all those involved with that person's care. Care must strive to be realistic and flexible, responding to the changing needs of an individual as their health deteriorates. For example, you may have a situation that involves someone with challenging behaviour, continued substance use, an uncertain illness trajectory and planning for end of life in a hostel setting. Utilising the MDT early on enables us to address current care needs and plan for future concerns in a way that is person-centred, not crisis led, thereby assisting practitioners to work safely. It is not enough for a person to have a service, but they need services to 'fit' them. Klop et al. (2018) encourage tailored solutions. Regular MDT meetings can support this individual approach to care.

Implications for policy and service development

The challenges raised in this chapter highlight the need for broad improvement of health and social care for this group, and system wide change to improve palliative care outcomes for PEHUS. To do this we must challenge the assumptions that people have a home within which they can (and want to be) cared for; that they have the support of friends and family around them; and we must champion ways of working that support people who may feel ambivalent towards their own health or lack the self-worth needed to enable them to access support.

New models of care need to be explored, utilising knowledge gained through research and practice in the field of inclusion health. These models could examine how the systemic barriers experienced by this group could be reduced; barriers such as zero tolerance policies around substance use, punitive action for 'non engagement' or difficult behaviour, fragmented clinical care and lack of joined up MDT working. In Table 9.6, we have outlined some examples of innovative models of care from our knowledge of practice that address these issues in different ways. They emphasise the need for flexibility to work with the uncertainty often found in these cases.

Conclusion

PEHUS do not receive equitable care as they approach the end of their lives. In trying to improve equity we must reflect on the lived experience of each individual and the challenges they face and understand how the services and systems involved in their care can often create and perpetuate barriers that exacerbate the multiple exclusion they already experience. Research (e.g. Shulman et al., 2018) tells us that homeless sector staff carry a heavy burden in supporting deteriorating health in hostel settings. Health and social care staff often have misconceptions about the level of support received in these environments, and needs are not always identified upon discharge from hospital.

While we have attempted to quantify this issue as we experience it and understand it from relevant research, we emphasise that any service or system change must be in response to local need.

We hope this chapter will encourage better partnership working on the ground, but also support upstream system change for broader and more sustainable transformations to take place. We hope that it will contribute to the much needed

Table 9.6 Examples of models of care to improve access to palliative care for PEHUS

Model	Description	Examples
Palliative care in-reach to hostel accommodation	Support from palliative care specialist offering advice and information on palliative issues to non-clinical homeless sector staff. Support can include education/training, attendance at case reviews, 1:1 case management support and advocacy.	Homeless Lead at St Luke's Hospice, Cheshire, UK Palliative Care Coordinator role at St Ann's Hospice, Manchester, UK St Luke's Hospice, Plymouth, UK
Specialist homeless hospice facility	24-hour nursing care facility offering a harm reduction approach to care, designed with needs and lifestyle of PEHUS in mind. The service offers flexible support to reflect the uncertainty of many illness trajectories, so people can remain in a familiar place as their health deteriorates. End-of-life patients accepted at these facilities.	Diane Morrison Hospice, Ottawa, Canada St Mungo's, London, UK
Palliative care street outreach programmes	Medical and palliative care provided on the street. Homeless outreach teams joined by palliative care professionals to engage and support entrenched rough sleepers. 'Street' acknowledged as a valid Preference for Place of Care and Death.	The PEACH (Palliative Education and Care for the Homeless) initiative. Toronto, Canada
Housing first	Provision of accommodation first for people experiencing homelessness, with wrap around to support for people once in stable accommodation. Reduction in barriers to good quality palliative care as experienced in standard hostel settings, e.g. medication storage, access, privacy.	Housing First England

discussions on this issue and empower the palliative care profession, current and future, and anyone working with homeless people using substances, to strive to work holistically and compassionately regardless of the complexity of the challenges faced.

For further reading on Inclusion Health standards please see Pathway: https://www.pathway.org.uk/wp-content/uploads/Version-3.1-Standards-2018-Final.pdf

References

Aldridge, R., Story, A., Hwang, S., Nordentoft, M., Luchenski, S., Hartwell, G., Tweed, E., Lewer, D., Vittal Katikireddi, S. and Hayward, A. (2018) 'Morbidity and mortality in homeless individuals, prisoners, sex workers, and individuals with substance use disorders in high-income countries: a systematic review and meta-analysis.' *The Lancet*, 391, pp. 241–250. DOI: 10.1016/S0140-6736(17)31869-X

Bell, J., Reed, K., Gross, S. and Witton, J. (2013) *The management of pain in people with a past or current history of addiction*. Salisbury, Action on Addiction. https://www.sldtraining.co.uk/media/i4clx50t/pain-management-in-those-with-addiction.pdf   [Accessed 15th March 2022].

Bramley, G. and Fitzpatrick, S. (2015) *Hard edges: mapping severe and multiple disadvantage in England*. Lankelly Chase Foundation. https://lankellychase.org.uk/wp-content/uploads/2015/07/Hard-Edges-Mapping-SMD-2015.pdf [Accessed 10th November 2021].

Cagle, J.G., Van Dussen, D.J., Culler, K.L., Carrion, I., Hong, S., Guralnik, J. and Zimmerman, S. (2014) 'Knowledge about hospice: exploring misconceptions, attitudes, and preferences for care.' *American Journal of Hospice and Palliative Care*, 33(1), pp. 27–33. DOI: 10.1177/1049909114546885

Cornes, M., Whiteford, M., Manthorpe, J. Neale, J., Byng, R., Hewett, N., Clark, M., Kilmister, A., Fuller, J., Aldridge, R. and Tinelli, M. (2018) 'Improving hospital discharge arrangements for people who are homeless: a realist synthesis of the intermediate care literature.' *Health and Social Care in the Community*, 26(3), pp. e345–e359. DOI: 10.1111/hsc.12474

Dolan, B. and Arnold, R. (2015) *Prognosis in decompensated chronic liver failure*. Fast facts and concepts #189, Palliative Care Network of Wisconsin. https://www.mypcnow.org/wp-content/uploads/2019/02/FF-189-prognosis-liver-failure.-3rd-Ed.pdf [Accessed 13th April 2022].

Fazel, S., Geddes, J.R. and Kushel, M. (2014) 'The health of homeless people in high-income countries: descriptive epidemiology, health consequences, and clinical and policy recommendations.' *Lancet*, 384(9953), pp. 1529–1540. DOI: 10.1016/S0140–6736(14)61132-6

Fazel, S., Khosla, V., Doll, H. and Geddes, J. (2008) 'The prevalence of mental disorders among the homeless in western countries: systematic review and meta-regression analysis.' *PLoS Medicine*, 5, p. e225. DOI: 10.1371/journal.pmed.0050225

Fitzpatrick, S., Bramley, G. and Johnsen, S. (2012) "Pathways into multiple exclusion homelessness in seven UK cities." *Urban Studies*, 50(1), pp. 148–168. DOI: 10.1177/0042098012452329

Galvani, S. (2018) *End of life care for people with alcohol and other drug problems: what we know and what we need to know. Final Project Report*. Manchester Metropolitan University. Available online at: http://e-space.mmu.ac.uk/622052/1/EOLC%20Final%20overview%20report%20 27%20November%202018%20PRINT%20VERSION.pdf [Accessed 4th March 2022].

Galvani, S. and Wright, S. (2019) Supporting people with substance problems at the end of life supporting people with substance problems at the end of life supporting people with substance problems at the end of life supporting people with substance problems at the end of life *Palliative and End of Life Care for People with Alcohol and Drug Problems (Policy Standards)*. Manchester, Manchester Metropolitan University. https://endoflifecaresubstanceuse.com/wp-content/uploads/2022/02/Policy-Standards-SU-and-EoLC-May-2019.pdf [Accessed 4th March 2022].

Galvani, S., Wright, S. and Witham, G. (2019) *Supporting people with substance problems at end of life (Good Practice Guidance)*. Manchester, Manchester Metropolitan University. https://endoflifecaresubstanceuse.com/wp-content/uploads/2022/02/Good-practice-guidance-EoLC-and-SU-April-2019-Web-version.pdf [Accessed 4th March 2022].

Hart, J.T. (1971) 'The inverse care law.' *The Lancet*, 297(7696), pp. 405–412. DOI: 10.1016/S0140-6736(71)92410-X

Homeless Palliative Care Toolkit. http://www.homelesspalliativecare.com/wp-content/uploads/2018/09/Questions-to-consider-tool.pdf [Accessed 8th May 2022].

Hospice UK. (2018) *Care committed to me*. London, Hospice UK. https://professionals.hospiceuk.org/docs/default-source/Policy-and-Campaigns/briefings-and-consultations-documents-and-files/care_committed_to_me_web.pdf?sfvrsn=0 [Accessed 13th April 2022].

Hudson, B.F., Fleming, K., Shulman, C. and Candy, B. (2016) 'Challenges to access and provision of palliative care for people who are homeless: a systematic review of qualitative research.' *BMC Palliative Care*, 15, pp. 1–18. DOI: 10.1186/s12904-016-0168-6

Klop, H.T., de Veer, A.J.E., van Dongen, S.I., Francke, A.L., Rietjens, J.A.C. and Onwuteaka-Philipsen, B.D. (2018) 'Palliative care for homeless people: a systematic review of the concerns, care needs and preferences, and the barriers and facilitators for providing palliative care.' *BMC Palliative Care*, 17(1), p. 67. DOI: 10.1186/s12904-018-0320-6. PMID: 29690870; PMCID: PMC5914070.

Leibowitz, L. and Krueger, J. (2013) 'Attitudes and stereotypes about the homeless: a study on self-persuasion and stereotype accuracy.' *Journal of Social Distress and the Homeless*, 14, pp. 3–4, pp. 125–150. DOI: 10.1179/sdh.2005.14.3–4.125

Luchenski, S., Maguire, N., Aldridge, R.W., Hayward, A., Story, A., Perri, P., Withers, J., Clint, S., Fitzpatrick, S. and Hewett, N. (2018) 'What works in inclusion health: overview of effective interventions for marginalised and excluded populations.' *Lancet* 391(10117), pp. 266–280. DOI: 10.1016/S0140–6736(17)31959-1

Maguire, N.J., Johnson, R., Vostanis, P., Keats, H. and Remington, R.E. (2009) *Homelessness and complex trauma: a review of the literature*. Southampton, UK. http://eprints.soton.ac.uk/id/eprint/69749 [Accessed 15th March 2022].

McCreaddie, M., Lyons, I., Watt, D., Ewing, E., Croft, J., Smith, M. and Tocher, J. (2010) 'Routines and rituals: a grounded theory of the pain management of drug users in acute care settings.' *Journal of Clinical Nursing*, 19(19–20), pp. 2730–2740. DOI: 10.1111/j.1365–2702.2010.03284.x

McNeil, R., Guirguis-Younger, M. and Dilley, L. (2012) 'Recommendations for improving the end-of-life care system for homeless populations: a qualitative study of the views of Canadian health and social services professionals.' *BMC Palliative Care*, 11, p. 14. http://www.biomedcentral.com/1472-684X/11/14Ryan [Accessed 15th March 2022].

McNeil, R., Guirguis-Younger, M. and Dilley, L. (2013) 'Learning to account for the social determinants of health affecting homeless persons.' *Medical Education*, 47(5), pp. 485–494. DOI: 10.1111/medu.12132

Office for National Statistics. (2020) *Deaths of homeless people in England and Wales: 2019 registrations*. ONS. [Online]. https://www.ons.gov.uk/peoplepopulationandcommunity/birthsdeathsandmarriages/deaths/bulletins/deathsofhomelesspeopleinenglandandwales/2019registrations [Accessed 15th March 2022].

Otis, J.D., Keane, T.M. and Kerns, R.D. (2003) 'An examination of the relationship between chronic pain and post-traumatic stress disorder.' *Journal of Rehabilitation Research & Development*, 40, pp. 397–405. DOI: 10.1682/JRRD.2003.09.0397

Prater, C.D., Zylstra, R.G. and Miller, K.E. (2002) 'Successful pain management for the recovering addicted patient.' *The Primary Care Companion to the Journal of Clinical Psychiatry*, 4(4), pp. 125–131. DOI: 10.4088/pcc.v04n0402

Public Health England. (2017) *Better care for people with co-occurring mental health and alcohol/drug use conditions.* London, PHE. https://assets.publishing.service.gov.uk/government/uploads/system/uploads/attachment_data/file/625809/Co-occurring_mental_health_and_alcohol_drug_use_conditions.pdf [Accessed 15th March 2022].

Purkey, E. and MacKenzie, M. (2019) 'Experience of healthcare among the homeless and vulnerably housed a qualitative study: opportunities for equity-oriented health care.' *International Journal of Equity Health*, 18, p. 101. DOI: 10.1186/s12939-019-1004-4

Queen, A.B., Lowrie, R., Richardson, J. and Williamson, A.E. (2017) 'Multimorbidity, disadvantage, and patient engagement within a specialist homeless health service in the UK: an in-depth study of general practice data.' *British Journal of General Practice Open*, 1(3). bjgpopen17X100941. DOI: 10.3399/bjgpopen17X100941

Rogans-Watson, R., Shulman, C., Lewer, D., Armstrong, M. and Hudson, B. (2020) 'Premature frailty, geriatric conditions and multimorbidity among people experiencing homelessness: a cross-sectional observational study in a London hostel.' *Housing, Care and Support*, 23(3/4), pp. 77–91. DOI: 10.1108/HCS-05-2020-0007

Royal College of Psychiatrists (RCPsych). (2018) *Our invisible addicts.* 2nd edition College Report CR211. London, Royal College of Psychiatrists. https://www.rcpsych.ac.uk/docs/-default-source/improving-care/better-mh-policy/college-reports/college-report-cr211.pdf?sfvrsn=820fe4bc_2 [Accessed 27th September 2021].

Shulman, C., Hudson, B., Kennedy, P., Brophy, N. and Stone, P. (2018) 'Evaluation of training on palliative care for staff working within a homeless hostel.' *Nurse Education Today*, 71, pp. 135–144. DOI: 10.1016/j.nedt.2018.09.022

Shulman, C., Hudson, B.F., Low, J., Hewett, N., Daley, J., Kennedy, P., Davis, S., Brophy, N., Howard, D., Vivat, B. and Stone, P. (2017) 'End of Life care for homeless people: a qualitative analysis exploring the challenges to access and provision of palliative care.' *Palliative Medicine*, pp. 36–45. DOI: 10.1177/0269216317717101

Thomas, B. (2012) *Homelessness kills: An analysis of the mortality of homeless people in early twenty-first century.* London, England, Crisis. https://www.crisis.org.uk/ending-homelessness/homelessness-knowledge-hub/health-and-wellbeing/homelessness-kills-2012/ [Accessed 15th March 2022].

Tobin, J., Rogers, A., Winterburn, I., Tullie, S., Kalyanasundaram, A., Kuhn, I. and Barclay, S. (2021) 'Hospice care access inequalities: a systematic review and narrative synthesis.' *BMJ Supportive & Palliative Care*, Published Online First: 19 February 2021. DOI: 10.1136/bmjspcare-2020–002719

Webb, W., Mitchell, T., Nyatanga, B. and Snelling, P. (2018) 'Nursing management of people experiencing homelessness at the end of life.' *Nursing Standard*, 32(27), pp. 53–63. DOI: 10.7748/ns.2018.e11070

Witham, G., Galvani, S. and Peacock, M. (2019a) 'End of life care for people with alcohol and drug problems: findings from a rapid evidence assessment.' *Health and Social Care Community*, 27(5), pp. e637–e650. DOI: 10.1111/hsc.12807

Witham, G., Yarwood, G., Wright, S. and Galvani, S. (2019b) 'An ethical exploration of the narratives surrounding substance use and pain management at the end of life: a discussion paper.' *Nursing Ethics*, 27(5). DOI: 10.1177/0969733019871685

10 Jane's journey

Substance use, palliative care and sex work

Adele Brien

Introduction

The aim of this chapter is to explore, through the use of a case study, the involvement and interventions of a Community Specialist Palliative Care Team in supporting a woman in her early 40s (who for confidentiality reasons we will call Jane) with lung cancer and spinal metastases who was also a sex worker and used substances. There is a paucity of literature and evidence related to end-of-life care and sex workers. We will aim to show how a multidisciplinary approach was essential to discover what Jane's priorities were, what was important to her and the best way we could meet her support needs while also gaining and keeping her trust and respect. This chapter will examine health inequalities for people in an urban inner city area, especially those marginalised in society such as sex workers and people with problematic substance use at the end of life. With specific reference to Jane, we will discuss the ways in which her social circumstances and lifestyle impacted her health and how her low expectations of what we could provide were managed in order to improve her care and experience of the whole multidisciplinary team.

We will explore the challenges and barriers related to caring for Jane including managing her medication, multiple symptoms and the impact of her 'partner' on the overall care she received throughout her journey. Jane continued working as a sex worker and using IV drugs until two weeks before her death.

Sex workers

According to Goldmann (2011), it is estimated that there are 40–42 million sex workers in the world of whom 75% are between 13 and 25 years old. They are a marginalised group in society, often limited to certain areas or neighbourhoods and tend to have multiple overlapping risk factors of morbidity/mortality, experiencing disproportionate social and health inequalities compared to the general population (Puri et al., 2017). A study by Haixia and Loke (2019) highlighted that female sex workers are stigmatised and marginalised around the world, not accepted in society and often labelled as immoral and troublemakers which can, at times, cause them to become excluded from the health sector.

DOI: 10.4324/9781003187882-13

There is a high degree of overlap between substance use and sex work (Luchenski et al., 2018). Puri et al. (2017) describe how becoming a sex worker often goes together with difficult life experiences such as family problems, childhood trauma, mental health, sexual abuse and drug dependence. Homelessness and drug dependence have been identified as two of the most significant factors which prompt engagement in street sex work and also two of the main barriers to stabilising the lives of street workers (Spice, 2007). Health inequalities are a significant problem with this group of people: they experience many occupational risks and are in need of multiple health services. Yet they face many difficulties accessing healthcare, and are often reluctant to engage with formal services, preferring to self-medicate (Struber et al., 2008). Stigma is possibly the biggest barrier to preventing sex workers from accessing health services and can be a major factor in increased risk of mental health problems, sexual health conditions, substance misuse and poor health in general (Rayson and Alba, 2019). It is critical that all health and social care workers critically examine their own beliefs in order to deliver non-judgemental and quality care to everyone.

The access that sex workers have to health services is a complex issue and health workers should take into account all the barriers which prevent this group of people from accessing healthcare, such as: opening hours, location and transport, patients' perceptions of services and expectations of what can be offered if they seek help. Women commonly experience social exclusion related to this occupation and are subject to socioeconomic disadvantages that can be detrimental to health; they can also have poor knowledge of their physical conditions and how to manage them (Polly et al., 2017). Their health risks, combined with limited perceptions of the seriousness of their health problems often lead to their main experience of healthcare being that of accessing emergency care in a crisis situation. In order to prevent this happening, we must create conditions to enable people to take control of their own lives and encourage them to have a voice. As discussed in the UK's Marmot review (2010), this is the only way to ensure that we as health professionals can focus on what matters to them.

Case study

Background

Jane was a 52-year-old woman who was referred to The Specialist Palliative Care Team by the Respiratory Specialist Nurse at the hospital. Her diagnosis was stage 4 lung cancer with cancer spread to the bones and adrenal glands. She had numerous other medical conditions which included chronic obstructive pulmonary disease, depression, arthritis and problematic substance use. Jane was experiencing pain and symptom management problems and had a history of non-concordance and poor attendance with appointments. She had previously been offered ten fractions of radiotherapy for back pain but had failed to attend the appointment several times and had been discharged from the hospital team. It was at this point that she was referred by the hospital Respiratory Specialist Nurse to the Community Palliative Care Team for specialist support. Although Jane was not accessing hospital services, the Specialist Nurse did not want Jane to be without any support in the community setting.

The only social background given to us on the referral was that Jane lived in a bedsit in a large, shared house and most of the other residents were taking drugs. The referral was processed and discussed at our daily triage meeting held with the whole Palliative Care Team to decide which clinician would be most appropriate for the patient, and it was decided that due to the environmental risks highlighted, clinicians would visit in pairs for their own safety. After several unsuccessful phone calls, a letter was sent offering Jane an initial home appointment and as she did not respond to the letter I visited the house on the date offered, hoping that I would get an answer at the property. Jane's partner (John) opened the main door and let me into the bedsit.

Initial assessment

Jane lived in a very small, untidy, dirty bedsit with John. It was accessed via communal stairs where numerous people were sitting, smoking and drinking. The bedsit consisted of a double bed and lots of bin bags scattered all over the room. There was no shower or bath and Jane was in a dirty nightdress with her hair matted into a knot on her head. John was present throughout the visit but made no effort to engage with me and 'slept' throughout the complete assessment. There was also another woman asleep on the floor at the bottom of the bed. Jane was very unkempt and weighed 45kg (seven stone). She reported she had no appetite and ate very little. I explained to Jane that she was at high risk of pressure damage and she allowed me to examine her body which highlighted a pressure ulcer on her bottom. She would later allow me to refer her to Community Nurses to manage the wound.

Jane informed me that she was afraid of living in the bedsit as other residents used drugs and homeless people slept in the stairwells at night. She also informed me that people would break into the room, threaten her and steal her money; and that she had been attacked several times when leaving the property. Jane was very erratic in taking pain medication and often took more than was prescribed – stating that these medications gave her no relief from the pain. After a thorough assessment it was decided that she needed stronger medication and a pain patch was prescribed (as it was safer than oral morphine due to risk of misuse). These were kept in a locked box in the bedsit, with only health professionals knowing the number to open the box and District Nurses would visit to apply the patch.

Sensitive conversations about substance use and sex work

Opioid misuse can be more common among patients with a history of illicit substance use (Ives et al., 2006), although at first assessment many deny any drug use, only feeling comfortable to disclose this once the practitioner has earnt their trust – which can take a considerable amount of time and numerous visits. This is related to stigma and is significant as without building the relationship and trust it can affect how we manage symptoms at the end of life (Witham et al., 2019).

Jane continually denied any drug use for many visits, despite there being syringes and foil wraps around the bedsit. She always stated they were her partner's, and although I explained that I was not there to stop her using drugs but to ensure I could prescribe safely around them, it took several weeks before she would open up about her life. Jane had been married, had one daughter and had worked as a receptionist in a brothel. She holidayed abroad twice a year and was very happy until her husband died and she became depressed. She lost her job, began drinking and met John who had a history of mental health problems and was a substance user. Over a period of time Jane became addicted to heroin and lost her home, she then moved into the bedsit. She informed me that she took heroin on a daily basis; she took as much as she could get – although the amount depended on the number of men who she had sex with. This was a major breakthrough as I could put safety measures (such as sharp bins) in the bedsit for any visiting healthcare professional and, with Jane's consent, share information with them and highlight this on any future referrals. It was essential from early in the relationship that I had a firm plan of action involving good communication, building trust and getting Jane's informed consent to share information in order for our relationship to work.

All clinicians in the Special Palliative Care Team have Advanced Communication skills which include recognising the importance of patient's cues and concerns (both verbal and nonverbal) and being very skilled in establishing relationships and building on from difficult conversations. This ensures that the patient is at the centre of each assessment and has more choice and control over their health and the way care is delivered – the importance of which is highlighted in both national and international policies (National Palliative and End of Life Care Partnership, 2015; Worldwide Palliative Care Alliance, 2014).

Advance care planning

Central to Advance Care Planning is that the wishes of the palliative patient are met and their preferences are known to all, both of which improve quality of life for people with life limiting illnesses (Mullick et al., 2013). In the case of people who are dependent on substances, advance care planning should also incorporate measures to prevent withdrawal. We spoke to other specialist agencies that could offer advice and support, and with Jane's consent we formulated a plan that involved substituting her heroin with oxycodone (which could be given either orally or subcutaneously), enabling Jane to avoid withdrawal episodes. Such multidisciplinary team working underpins good patient centred care: establishing good working relationships with partner agencies helps to ensure consistent care across different healthcare settings, improving flexibility and responsiveness to meet outcomes that matter to patients (Gayle et al., 2013).

The Specialist Dietician and I initiated joint visits and established a mutually trusting relationship with Jane, which eventually led to some open and honest conversations. She began to be more honest about her circumstances, which enabled Jane to receive a lot of practical support (such as a grant to help her buy bedding and directing her to local foodbanks), but also a lot of psychological input from both myself and the dietician. This involved reassuring Jane that we would try our best to manage any pain and symptom problems and also to ensure that her choices were met wherever possible.

When John was present the visits were usually over quite quickly as Jane did not talk much. But if John was out, Jane would tell us stories about her daughter and show us photographs of her on holidays before she became a substance user and sex worker. By working with the dietician Jane began taking supplement drinks to provide her with much needed essential nutrients for her body. These were prescribed on a weekly basis as it is common for these to be sold to other drug users or used in place of any food to save money to spend on drugs. Indeed, it became a regular occurrence for Jane's partner to ring the team claiming the drinks had not arrived or had been stolen in order to get further supply. We were aware we were being manipulated in this way and tried to control this as much as possible, but it was still essential to supply these drinks to Jane and hope she was taking some of them as prescribed.

Over many visits Jane began to open up even more to me, sharing personal information. When alone she discussed how John would persuade her to have sex with men to earn money to fund their drug habit. Although she hated it, she would not let me intervene to find her a place of safety away from him. Jane appeared to be fiercely loyal to John and believed he was the one looking after her and keeping her safe. Collinson et al. (2011) suggest that although to the outside world it may appear that the partner is a pimp, closer examination of the relationship may suggest that sex work can be attributed to altruism rather than coercion. In addition, Collinson et al. (2011) describe how many sex workers were worried to take up any help or services as it may mean leaving their partner behind, which they did not want to do. On reflection, this evidence seemed to describe Jane's relationship with John because although she said she hated what she was doing, she seemed to think it was her responsibility to earn money for them both to buy drugs and the only way this seemed to be able to be remedied was by removing Jane from this situation. Although this way of living was unsafe, Jane had full capacity to make these decisions. We had to respect that and help her in any way she allowed us to, ensuring we did not make any judgements that would ruin the relationship we had already built.

Palliative treatment and care

Throughout our time working with and caring for Jane she had experienced radiating back pain which was concerning because of her high risk of spinal cord compression. One fraction of radiotherapy was offered, and I accompanied Jane to the hospital for the radiotherapy. Jane's anxieties were not related to the actual procedure but what the other people in the waiting room and the health professionals' opinion of her would be. By this point she was very emaciated and her hair was still knotted and mangled. The radiotherapy went ahead and over time helped ease the pain.

The health and wellbeing of sex workers is unfortunately hindered by social stigma: negative labelling marginalises their position in society, resulting in their needs being unmet and increasing health inequalities (Sanders et al., 2009). Interviews with sex workers carried out by Mellor and Lovell (2012) found that some of the main barriers to accessing services were: negative attitudes of staff in relation to patient drug use and lifestyle; the women's embarrassment about their lives, and a lack of knowledge about what was available and how to access the services. The women interviewed had low expectations regarding health care and appeared to disengage quickly, failing to keep appointments or develop a relationship with the health professionals. Studies carried out by both Ma et al. (2017) and Jeal et al. (2017) exploring street sex workers' views towards drug treatment also highlighted that they felt unable to disclose their sex work in attempts to prevent themselves from being stigmatised.

The impact of social disapproval can be especially significant if it comes from health professionals who have decision-making power over health interventions, treatment and care. Such professional stigmatisation may involve labelling and stereotyping and can often stop people from seeking help from organisations (Benoit et al., 2015). Yet what became apparent with Jane was how she had also developed high levels of self-stigma: only accepting help when her symptoms became unmanageable and she was in a crisis situation. By the time she was seen by the Community Palliative Care Team, she had missed numerous hospital appointments and avoided interaction with healthcare workers as much as possible.

Sadly, this is a reoccurring problem that palliative care teams face, as the referral is often only made when all other lines of help have been exhausted. This is why a thorough assessment and identification of needs is essential in the continuing care of a patient, to engage the patient, encourage them to be active in their own care and help them feel they have some control over their life.

Continuous, non-judgemental support

I visited Jane several times a week when I could gain access to her bedsit. This remained problematic throughout the whole journey, as there would be occasions when no one answered the door. One several occasions, when I arrived on the street, I would see Jane buying drugs and this was usually the time of the no access visits. I never told Jane I saw her or why I thought I could not gain access, as I did not want her to think I was judging her.

John was usually present when I did gain access and Jane did not appear to want to speak about the future in front of him. But on one visit several months into me supporting her, Jane was alone and I took the opportunity to ask what was important to her and if she had any plans or wishes as her health deteriorated. I ensured that I shared information and discussed plans at a level that Jane understood so she did not become overwhelmed. This was assessed by asking Jane to share what she understood of her illness and listening to the language she used.

Shiffman et al. (2011) highlight how crucial this is, reporting that patients did not engage well if they did not understand the information given to them. Jane would often share that she felt in the past healthcare staff had not involved her in decision-making but made decisions around her. This was also highlighted by Templeton et al. (2018) who discussed the importance of using a holistic approach that includes family, friends and carers to address the complex issues and work effectively in a compassionate and skilful manner.

Jane and I continued advance care planning over several weeks and engaged in very frank conversations in relation to her home circumstances and her relationship with John. Jane confided in me that she felt dirty and was very disappointed with herself for the way her life had turned out. Jane did not have regular contact with her daughter (or granddaughter) since she found out her mum was having sex with men to pay for drugs. Despite this Jane would not allow me to put a safeguarding measure in or try to move her away from John. This appeared to be fuelled by both her dependence on drugs and her loyalty to John. This type of relationship is discussed by Fox and Galvani (2020) describing how substances may be used within a relationship as a form of bonding but also can be used to control a partner through limiting access to substances or supplying substances in a way that makes separating more complex.

Jane and I discussed what would happen as her health and wellbeing deteriorated in this environment and she agreed that it would not be a nice place to die. It would be very difficult to manage end of life medication in the home due to her vulnerability and the people visiting the flat. Together we explored other options open to her – including hospices – and I offered to refer her to the hospice for a short period of time to assess her pain and to allow her to see if this may be somewhere she would consider for end-of-life care.

Jane's main concern regarding hospice admission was the heroin withdrawal process. So I spoke to a drug and alcohol team and a plan was formulated on how to stop the withdrawal symptoms by using oral liquid morphine. This was explained to Jane and she was brave enough to agree to try this following admission to the hospice. Despite resistance from John who was adamant that he could look after Jane better than anyone and that she should stay at home, I worked with a local hospice who agreed to accept my referral of Jane and she was admitted there a few days later.

Hospice care

On the day of admission I received a call from the ambulance who had arrived to pick Jane up. They asked if I could speak to her as they found her wandering up and down the street approaching men offering them sex. Jane told me she was trying to get some money for John before she left as he would not have any money coming in while she was away. I managed to convince Jane to stop this and she agreed to get into the ambulance.

I visited several times at the hospice and the change in her appearance was remarkable. She was clean and her hair had been washed and brushed; she had also begun to eat properly. She informed me that she did not want to take heroin again and was either going to live at her daughter's or move into a flat alone if she was offered one on discharge. Notably Jane told me she had not felt this good in years. Jane was still adamant she would not return back to the flat and on the condition that she remained clean of drugs, her daughter invited her to move in with her. Following three weeks of hospice stay, she was discharged to her daughter's care. Jane was very proud that she had not taken any drugs at this time and would mention this regularly.

About two weeks after moving in with her daughter, Jane returned to the flat to see John and never returned to her daughters. The drug taking and sex work began again. Following regular visits from me, Jane was admitted to hospital where she was diagnosed with sepsis. Unfortunately, due to her drug dependence, she self-discharged herself home two days later – before treatment could be finished.

Jane continued to deteriorate rapidly, she was doubly incontinent and hallucinating. Despite this there still appeared to be several men waiting outside the door to have sex with her and I felt it was essential that I advocate for Jane to remove her from that environment. I told her she was now approaching the end of her life and that the time had come to go back into the hospice before she was too unwell to be moved. She agreed, the hospice accepted her straight away and that day she was readmitted.

On both admissions to the hospice, Jane had a Sexually Transmitted Infection (STI) and received treatment for this. Although research suggests condom use has increased over the last 30 years (Scambler and Paoli, 2008), STIs remain an inevitable risk among street workers. While there are agencies that help street workers, the women need to access this help. I had contacted one of those agencies previously, who informed me that Jane was well known to them and despite being very frail, was a regular attender on the streets in the local area most nights. But she did not engage with them most of the time.

During Jane's admission John visited regularly and was often verbally aggressive to the staff. He would take her into the garden in a wheelchair and staff had observed him trying to give her drugs. He also tried to take her home on one occasion and this resulted in the hospice staff banning him from visiting again for Jane's safety. This is not unique to this case study. Galvani et al. (2018) found similar experiences with hospice staff highlighting concerns regarding misuse of drugs and medication. Ware et al. (2021) also found similar staff concerns about people using substances and their families, commonly relating to family discord, higher medication being requested and reluctance to allow medication monitoring.

Two weeks later Jane died peacefully at the hospice where she was safe and clean, with her daughter present. I continued to visit Jane at the hospice until her death.

Discussion

The aim of this discussion section is to distil some of the general principles in my work with Jane, to highlight the professional approach that can be translated into working with other patients. At Jane's initial assessment it was important to allow her to identify what she felt were the most important issues to her at that time and share information she felt comfortable to tell me, but not to pressure her for information she was not willing to give to a 'stranger'. Each visit that followed consisted of building mutual trust to help her realise the importance of full disclosure about her life in order to help her take ownership of her health needs. All healthcare professionals need to endeavour to leave any preconceived ideas, stereotypes and judgements behind them. In Jane's case, if she wanted to discuss her life I would listen, but I needed to remember that her current situation was only a small part of who Jane was as a person and should not impact at all on the care she received.

Good symptom management is essential, although it was difficult to achieve due to Jane's use of illicit drugs (mainly heroin on a daily basis). It became apparent early on that certain oral medication could be abused and possibly misused by others if prescribed because the bedsit was used by many people throughout a day. Therefore flawless multidisciplinary team working between the palliative care team, District Nurses and the General Practitioner (GP) was essential. As part of this, it was decided that although I am an independent prescriber, there should be only one prescriber in Jane's care and this should be the GP. It is extremely important when assessing a patient with substance dependence to build up a comprehensive understanding of their substance use to help identify and manage risks, address coexisting social problems, and deliver effective harm reducing interventions. It was essential that Jane receive the medication she needed, but also crucial that the Multi Disciplinary Team (MDT) could monitor the risk of abuse.

The principles of pain control for people using substances are no different to other patients needing treatment, although they may lack the skills to follow regimes with oral medication and their ability to attend follow up appointments may be compromised. There are also likely to be psychological, social and existential issues that influence pain and behaviour, such as the feeling of being judged and losing faith in the health profession. It is therefore helpful for the multidisciplinary team to look beyond the substance use to its causes and implications. In this context, the expectations of both patient and nurse can be different and the interaction can be equally frustrating for both. This is why at each assessment it is essential for the nurse to lay out the boundaries with the patient, allowing the nurse to offer clear advice on what are realistic expectations. This also involves what cannot be achieved with levels of prescribing that may need to be higher for substance users due to their tolerance to opioids even if this may contravene clinical guidelines in relation to opioid titration (Carmichael et al., 2016). Frankness and honesty are usually well accepted within this marginalised group, although tolerance is needed between both parties, the willingness to accept the opinion or behaviour of others despite not agreeing with it is essential. It is also very important not to promise or offer things that may not be available (such as ongoing monetary funds), as this could be detrimental to the trust element of the relationship between the patient and the healthcare professional.

Jane was living in extreme social deprivation. She was very embarrassed about her living conditions which was why she had not accepted any help from outside agencies for her healthcare or her housing issues. As discussed by Mellor and Lovell (2012), it is very common for women belonging to this marginalised group to become socially excluded and their chaotic circumstances often obscure understanding of the seriousness of their health problems. This can result in a delay in accessing help which often only occurs in response to a crisis. This may be due to a combination of substance use supressing health symptoms so they are overlooked; not understanding the seriousness of the health problem but also the pressure to make money to fund drug use which can become the main priority. All of this this can make things very difficult for the practitioner as they only have a short period of time to gain the trust of the patient and advance care plan before their health begins to deteriorate.

In critically unpacking Jane's story, the key questions related to her health are articulated in Table 10.1. The problems she faced were complex and multifaceted, requiring effective communication skills and an appreciation of the wider social and economic factors that impacted on her life.

Dignity and choice are essential for good end-of-life care, and it is important that every patient has a good quality of life and that their pain and symptoms are managed up until their death. This involves identifying people in the last phase of their life and having conversations about their wishes and choices to facilitate good, personalised care. Jane needed a designated care co-ordinator to bring together a multidisciplinary team that, working together would ensure she received the best care. It became my role to advocate for her to enable she received dignity at the end of her life. The most important thing was that Jane had choice and the opportunity to prepare for her death.

Conclusion

Marginalised groups are often described as hard to reach, although from their perspective it is frequently supportive and non-judgemental services that are hard to reach. Research on sex workers and palliative/end-of-life care is very limited at present, and a more comprehensive evidence base is needed to build good future policy and practice both in the United Kingdom and internationally. This chapter has drawn largely on the practical experience of working with people using substances, using a case study to draw out key learning for healthcare professionals.

More research is also needed to investigate barriers to health services: how we as health professionals can engage earlier with palliative patients to prevent it becoming a crisis situation; and how to encourage this marginalised group of people to seek out help earlier without feeling judged. All patients deserve non-judgemental and compassionate care that meets their individual needs and ensures their wishes are met wherever possible. Yet this marginalised group does not appear to be receiving the same level of service as other people at the end of their life, as highlighted in my own professional experience where breaking down barriers requires a lot of work and time.

Table 10.1 Key questions/challenges and good practice

Key questions	Challenges	Good practice
How do I gain information from patients about their health?	Patient may be reluctant to give full disclosure due to substance use and life circumstances.	Building mutual trust takes time. Patients may have had past negative experiences of professionals and stigma.
How do I ensure good symptom management for the patient?	Patient may be reluctant to admit their substance use history or may give incorrect information on substance use.	Practitioners need to remember that patients may need higher ranges of prescribing doses due to tolerance of opioids. Having only one prescriber within an MDT prevents attempts to get multiple prescriptions across different health professionals.
How do I ensure social deprivation does not impact the quality of healthcare service provided?	Patient may be reluctant to engage with other health or palliative care providers due to personal, environmental circumstances.	Working within a multi-disciplinary team and introducing other team members as joint visits will enable the patient to begin to trust professionals as they may have had bad experiences in the past when trying to access services.
How do I try to ensure patients choices and wishes are met wherever possible?	Patient may feel they have no choices due to circumstances and may not trust people enough to open up to advance care planning.	Spend time listening to the patient and build trust so they are able to discuss their choices. Advance care plan from the first visit and continue to do this throughout the patient's journey. Ensure all other services know of these plans.

A more proactive way of increasing engagement of marginalised groups with services is needed, taking into account the difficulties that sex workers have engaging and trusting healthcare workers without feeling judged. This could be improved by forging links with other services for women who sell sex and working together as a larger multidisciplinary team to meet specialist health and social care needs.

Communication and the attitudes of health and care staff have a significant impact on patients and their end-of-life care. The fear of being judged is stopping marginalised groups from seeking help until it becomes an emergency. This makes good end-of-life care difficult as sufficient time is required to understand what is important to the individual patient and what their expectations are, in order to allow for good advance care planning. Any personal judgements need to be cast aside to ensure no negative stereotyping or discriminatory behaviours are taking place. Only when this happens across all health and social care services will this marginalised group of people receive the care they need. Ultimately more work is needed with this growing group of people to ensure good care and equal access to services.

References

Benoit, C., McCarthy, B. and Jansson, M. (2015) 'Stigma, sex work and substance use: a comparative analysis.' *Sociology of Health and Illness*, 37(3), pp. 437–451. DOI: 10.1111/1467-9566.12201

Carmichael, A., Morgan, L. and Fabbro, E. (2016) 'Identifying and assessing the risk of opioid abuse in patients with cancer: an integrative review.' *Substance Abuse and Rehabilitation*, 7, pp. 71–79. DOI: 10.2147/SAR.S85409

Collinson, S., Straub, R. and Perry, G. (2011) 'The invisible men: finding and engaging with the male partners of street workers.' *Journal of Men's Health*, 8(3), pp. 202–207. DOI: 10.1016/j.jomh.2011.03.008

Fox, S. and Galvani, S. (2020) *Substance use and domestic abuse – essential information for social workers*. The British Association of Social Workers. https://www.basw.co.uk/system/files/resources/substance-use-and-domestic-abuse-pocket-guide.pdf   [Accessed 11th March 2022].

Galvani, S., Dance, C. and Wright, S. (2018) *Experiences of hospice and substance use professionals: end of life care for people with alcohol and drug problems*. Manchester, Manchester Metropolitan University. https://endoflifecaresubstanceuse.com/wp-content/uploads/2018/11/end-of-life-care-for-people-with-substance-use-professionals-perspective-full-report.pdf [Accessed 15th March 2022].

Gayle, N., Health, G., Cameron, E., Rashid, S. and Redwood S. (2013) 'Using the framework method for the analysis of qualitative data in multidisciplinary health research.' *BMC Medicine Research Methodology*, 13, p. 117. DOI: 10.1186/1471-2288-13-117

Goldmann, C. (2011) *Current assessment of the state of prostitution: recognise, understand and fight sexual exploitation*. 3rd Edition, Foundation Scelles. https://www.fondations-celles.org/pdf/current-assessment-of-the-state-of-prostitution-2013.pdf. [Accessed 10th March 2022].

Haixia, M. and Loke, A.Y. (2019) 'A qualitative study on female sex workers experience of stigma in the health care setting in Hong Kong.' *International Journal for Equity in Health*, 18(1), pp. 1–14. DOI: 10.1186/s12939-019-1084-1

Ives, T.J., Chelminski, P.R., Hammett-Stabler, C.A., Malone, R.M., Perhac, S.J., Potisek, N.M., Shilliday, B.B., Dewalf, D.A. and Pignone, M.P. (2006) 'Predictors of opioid misuse in patients with chronic pain: a prospective cohort study.' *BMC Health Services Research*, 6(46). DOI: 10.1186/1472-6963-6-46

Jeal, N., Macleod, J., Salisbury, C. and Turner, K. (2017) 'Identifying possible reasons why female street sex workers have poor drug treatment outcomes: a qualitative study.' *BMJ Open*, 7, p. e013018. DOI: 10.1136/bmjopen-2016-013018

Luchenski, S., Maguire, N., Aldridge, R.W. and Hayward, A. (2018) 'What works in inclusion health: overview of effective intervention for marginalised and excluded population.' *The Lancet*, 391, pp. 266–280. DOI: 10.1016/S0140-6736(17)31959-1

Ma, P., Chan, Z. and Loke, A. (2017) 'The socio-ecological model approach to understanding barriers and facilitators to the accessing of health services by sex workers: a systematic review.' *Aids and Behaviour*, 21(8), pp. 2412–2438. DOI: 10.1007/s10461-017-1818-2

Marmot Review Team. (2010) *Fair society, healthy lives: review of health inequalities in England post-2010*. London, The Marmot Review Team.

Mellor, R. and Lovell, A. (2012) 'The lived experiences of UK street based sex workers and the health consequences: an exploratory study.' *Health Promotion International*, 3, pp. 311–322. DOI: 10.1093/heapro/dar040

Mullick, A., Martin, J. and Sallnow, L. (2013) 'An introduction to advance care planning in practice.' *British Medical Journal*, 347, p. f6064. DOI: 10.1136/bmj.f6064

National Palliative and End of Life Care Partnership. (2015) *Ambitions for palliative and end of life care, national framework for local action*. https://acpopc.csp.org.uk/system/files/documents/2021-05/FINAL_Ambitions-for-Palliative-and-End-of-Life-Care_2nd_edition.pdf [Accessed 10th March 2022].

Polly, H., Zenobia, C. and Loke, A. (2017) 'The socio-ecological model approach to understanding barriers and facilitators to the accessing of health services by sex workers: A systematic review.' *Aids and Behaviour*, 21(8), pp. 2412–2438. DOI: 10.1007/s10461-017-1818-2

Puri, N., Shannon, K., Ngyen, P. and Goldenberg, S. (2017) 'Burden and correlations of mental health diagnosis among sex workers in an urban setting.' *Women's Health*, 17(1), p. 133. DOI: 10.1186/s12905-017-0491-y

Rayson, J. and Alba, B. (2019) 'Experiences of stigma and discrimination as predictors of mental health help seeking among sex workers.' *Sexual and Relationship Therapy*, 34(3), pp. 277–289. DOI: 10.1080/14681994.2019.1628488

Sanders, T., O'Neill, M. and Pitcher, J. (2009) *Prostitution: sex work, policy and politics*. London, Sage Publications.

Scambler, G. and Paoli, F. (2008) 'Health work, female sex workers and HIV/AIDS: global dimensions of stigma and deviance as barriers to interventions.' *Social Science & Medicine*, 66(8), pp. 1848–1862. DOI: 10.1016/j.socscimed.2008.01.002

Shiffman, S., Gerlach, K.K., Sembower, M.A. and Rohay, J.M. (2011) 'Consumer understanding of prescription drug information: An illustration using an antidepressant medication.' *Annals of Pharmacotherapy*, 45(4), pp. 452–458. DOI: 10.1345/aph.1P477

Spice, W. (2007) 'Management of sex workers and other high risk groups.' *Occupational Medicine*, 57, pp. 322–328. DOI: 10.1093/occmed/kqm045

Struber, J., Meyer, I. and Link, B. (2008) 'Stigma, prejudice, discrimination and health.' *Social Science & Medicine*, 67(3), pp. 351–357. DOI: 10.1016/j.socscimed.2008.03.023

Templeton, L., Yarwood, G., Wright, S. and Galvani, S. (2018) *Experiences of families, friends and carers: end of life care for people with alcohol and drug problems*. Research briefing No 4. Manchester, Manchester Metropolitan University. https://endoflifecaresubstanceuse.com/wp-content/uploads/2018/08/family-strand-briefing-31-july-2018-final.pdf [Accessed 10th March 2022].

Ware, O., Cagle, J., McPherson, M., Sacco, P., Frey, J. and Guralnik, J. (2021) 'Confirmed medication diversion in hospice care: qualitative findings from a sample of agencies.' *Journal of Pain and Symptom Management*, 61(4), pp. 789–796. DOI: 10.1016/j.jpainsymman.2020.09.013

Witham, G., Yarwood, G., Wright, S. and Galvani, S. (2019) 'An ethical exploration of the narratives surrounding substance use and pain management at the end of life: a discussion paper.' *Nursing Ethics*, 27(5), pp. 1344–1354. DOI: 10.1177/0969733019871685

Worldwide Palliative Care Alliance. (2014) *Global atlas of palliative care at end of life*. https://www.who.int/nmh/Global_Atlas_of_Palliative_Care.pdf [Accessed 10th March 2022].

11 Reflecting on the challenges and inequalities facing Black and minoritized communities in accessing substance use services, palliative and end-of-life care

Anya Ahmed and Lorna Chesterton

Introduction

There is now a deep divide in the United Kingdom (UK) between those who have and those who have not (Marmot, 2010, 2020) with continuing austerity measures and cuts to welfare affecting those already living in poverty the most (Duffy, 2012). Consequentially 14.5 million people live below the poverty line, with Black and minoritized households being twice as likely to live in poverty and three times as likely to experience persistent poverty (Social Metrics Commission, 2020). Compounding these factors are discrimination, marginalization and social exclusion (Bhopal, 2014), which can be linked to ethnicity, religion, culture and stigma. These layers of inequality become the foundations for poor health, poor health literacy and limited opportunities. In addition, poverty, poor housing and low educational attainment increase the risk of deprivation-related behaviours such as substance use, alcohol use (Caldwell et al., 2008) and tobacco smoking (Casetta et al., 2017). Areas of deprivation are also known to have less community service provision, more shops selling alcohol (Jones et al., 2015) and be an environment where drug markets thrive (UKDP, 2010). Deprived areas have the highest rates of illicit opiate and/or crack cocaine use (most specifically in the north of England) which also have the poorest treatment outcomes (Black, 2020). Additionally, it has been reported that a disproportionate number of deaths from substance use poisoning occur in deprived areas (Black, 2020) and that people in those areas experience the most severe impact from alcohol misuse (Public Health England, 2016).

The chapter will provide a brief overview of the complex challenges facing Black and minoritized communities in the UK. Throughout the chapter, we will use the term 'Black and minoritized' and highlight the heterogeneity of this population group. Following this, we will discuss substance use and end-of-life care as discrete areas of research, drawing on the cultural and religious attitudes surrounding them. We will then use an intersectional approach to explore how multiple layers of disadvantage and discrimination overlap and compound one another using case studies which are derived from our experience in practice.

DOI: 10.4324/9781003187882-14

Population diversity in the UK

Individuals identifying as being from a Black and minoritized background account for 14.4% of the UK population (UK Parliament, 2020). Within this population there is further diversity which is often masked by a generic description of a vague geographic region, such as South Asian, which may mean that a person is from one of a number of countries (e.g. Afghanistan, Bangladesh, India, Pakistan). Even specific reference to place of origin does not signify homogeneity, as there may be differences between generations or in people's social situation. It would, therefore, be problematic to assume that all individuals from a certain group were going to have the same beliefs and values (Calanzani et al., 2013). Moreover, minoritized groups also encompass individuals identifying as Irish, LGBTQ+, Gypsy, Roma and Traveller communities.

The ageing demographic of people from Black and minoritized communities, intersects with two main areas of knowledge. First, that older people from these population groups will be negatively impacted by health inequalities across their life course as they are more likely to live in deprived areas (Kings Fund, 2020) and as a result have lower life expectancy and poorer health in older age (Marmot, 2020). Second, that Black and minoritized populations are under-represented in service provision, for alcohol and substance use (Bayley and Hurcombe, 2011) and palliative and end-of-life care (Care Quality Commission (CQC), 2016). Such lack of engagement and access with both these services has far-reaching effects on individuals and their families, resulting in unmet needs, reduced quality of life and the loss of opportunities for advanced care planning (Aldridge and Bradley, 2017).

Alcohol and other drug use

Statistically, White British people make up 84% of those receiving help for drug and alcohol problems in England, with a further 5% from other White groups, with no other ethnic group representing more than 1% of those receiving treatment (Public Health England, 2020). Despite these figures, the UK police continue to target individuals from Black and minoritized backgrounds using 'stop and search' methods, which show, for instance, that Black people are nine times more likely to be stopped and three times more likely to be arrested than White people (Home Office, 2020). This leads us to conclude that while drug prevalence is higher among White people, they are at less risk of being suspected or arrested by the police in comparison to those from Black and minoritized backgrounds (Askew and Salinas, 2019). Such racial disparity and structural racism create false stereotypes, exacerbate stigma and further marginalization for communities, while embedding a mistrust of organizational systems from people within minoritized communities (Alexander, 2012). The United Nations Human Rights Council (2021: 8) described the UK as a place where 'minorities are disproportionately impacted in terms of arrest, pretrial detention, and conviction rates'.

When appraising literature around substance use in Black and minoritized groups this is generally broken down into specific religious groups or ethnicity. A study by Taak et al. (2021) looked at alcohol use in UK Punjabi-Sikh communities and discussed the conflicting religious tenets and the social acceptability of alcohol. Exploring substance use in this population group presents an interesting dichotomy since the Sikh religion prohibits alcohol, smoking and substance use while the Punjabi community has historically socially situated the heavy drinking cultures of men in terms of gendered masculinity (Oliffe et al., 2010). It is also apparent that sociocultural beliefs and attitudes can change over generations as communities are influenced by Western culture, a situation observed by Motune (2011) who reports a rising use of alcohol, particularly in second-generation Sikh women. However, Galvani et al. (2013) observed that while Westernized culture can influence younger people to become involved in drinking, it also afforded them knowledge of the effects of drinking.

It is relatively recently that research on drug and alcohol use for those identifying as Muslims in both Muslim-majority and Muslim-minority countries has emerged (Manickam et al., 2014; Mauseth et al., 2016). This is no doubt due to the fact that the Muslim religion prohibits the use of alcohol and drugs (Ali-Northcott, 2013) with scripture promoting a healthy lifestyle (Aboul-Enein, 2016). Such rules have created a culture which stigmatizes alcohol and drug use and users making it difficult for people to access services (Mallik et al., 2021). Evidence suggests that there is a particular stigma and strong prohibition and policing by families around women using alcohol (Valentine et al., 2010). This also reflects the stricter rules governing women's bodies and identities, within specific communities (Valentine et al., 2009).

The Polish community make up one of the largest sections of non-British citizens, with a population totalling 738,000 (Office for National Statistics, 2020). Evidence suggests increasing alcohol use and alcohol-related harm and drug use in this community, linked to increased risk of depression and suicide (Thom, et al., 2010). Maciagowska and Hanley (2017) reported that male Polish migrants were reluctant to access treatment services for alcohol and drug use, with Thickett and Bayley (2013) suggesting that this was due to services being culturally inappropriate. A study by Gleeson et al. (2020) explored the experiences of Polish women in the UK and their alcohol use and access to treatment, finding social sanctions and dependence upon male support could mean that the problematic use of alcohol in this population group is under-estimated. Despite the size of the Polish community in the UK, this population group remains an under-researched group, especially where alcohol and drug use are concerned (Gleeson et al., 2020).

The literature also shows that people from Black and minoritized communities are under-represented in alcohol and drug use services (Bayley and Hurcombe, 2011) and in mental health services (Memon et al., 2016). This reluctance to engage with services may reflect the stigma and religious prohibition, which is seen in many cultures, forcing individuals to conceal problems from the family and community (Bayley and Hurcombe, 2011). Other barriers include: a lack of awareness around alcohol use, language barriers, limited knowledge of services (Gleeson et al., 2019) and cultural attitudes towards help-seeking behaviour (Taak et al., 2021). This picture of under-representation is also observed in the majority population in the UK, where it is estimated that five out of six people who are alcohol dependent are failing to access services (Gleeson et al., 2019). However, it is also documented that ethnicity and community can act as a safeguard and protective mechanism against drug use, with studies suggesting that numbers are low from Black and minoritized communities because of religious restrictions and family ties which reduce the incidence and prevalence of drug use (Hurcombe et al., 2010). Thus, it could be argued that the informal networks present in many Black and minoritized communities could benefit from knowledge and skill sharing within those structures.

Black and minoritized groups are under-represented in drug and alcohol services for numerous reasons, such as family ties and cultural beliefs, but most worryingly from structural inequalities. Changing our focus to look at palliative and end-of-life care, it is interesting to observe if similar challenges and barriers are present.

Palliative and end-of-life care provision for individuals from the Black and minoritized communities

The term palliative care encompasses the journey from diagnosis to end-of-life care, and beyond, to bereavement after death (Meier et al., 2011). While palliative care has been freely available for decades in the UK, evidence suggests that Black and minoritized groups are under-represented in these services (Dixon et al., 2018) a situation which is apparent across most healthcare provision (King's Fund, 2021). The reason for such absences can be observed in the homogeneous nature of palliative services in terms of their structure, composition, settings and services which ignores the diversity of the population (Smith et al., 2013). Indeed, Cain et al. (2018) comment that a person's culture will influence individual's decisions around treatment and care, patterns of communication, and the quality of life and suffering, both during illness and at end of life. The literature also shows that individuals from Black and minoritized backgrounds have poorer experiences when they access end-of-life services (Dixon et al., 2018).

It is estimated that by 2026, 1.3 million people aged over 65 and 0.5 million people over 70 will be from Black and minoritized backgrounds in the UK (Koffman, 2018). Such diversity brings with it religious and cultural differences which influence health seeking behaviours and attitudes towards illness (Calanzani et al., 2013), both of which need to be reflected in service design. Certainly, there is an underlying Christian ethos in the UK Hospice movement and this inference continues as hospices often adopt the names of Christian saints which may have an exclusionary influence on non-Christians. Indeed, the conceptualization of what defines a 'good death' itself derives from Western ethics (Hart et al., 1998).

In today's diverse society, many people believe illnesses to be 'acts of God', which can sometimes mean that treatment options seem at odds with faith. This can be particularly apparent when dealing with a terminal prognosis, which may appear to be renouncing faith in God's power to sustain life (Wicher and Meeker, 2012). The literature demonstrates that cultural beliefs and values fundamentally impact people's perceptions around death, dying and decision making in end-of-life care (e.g. Kim et al. 2010). Certainly, all cultures have affective systems around death, whereby social processes articulate the norms around thinking and feeling about death and dying (Richards and Krawczyk, 2021). With a person's cultural beliefs contributing towards the meaning and importance of illness (Worster et al., 2018). Indeed, dying was once seen as being entirely the preserve of the church. In recent times it has moved to the preserve of medical science, which now aims to preserve life and avoid death, thus removing it from God's will (Howarth, 2007). There is also evidence that service providers assume that families from minority backgrounds wish to care for 'their own' (Calanzani et al., 2013).Such assumptions and cultural generalizations can, according to Harries et al. (2019), directly impact health and social care provision for older people from Black and minoritized backgrounds. However, cultural ideas around death and dying may change as second- and third-generation migrants adopt a more Westernized perspective (Parkes et al., 2015).

Thus far, we have focussed on the separate relationships between Black and marginalized groups and substance use and palliative/end-of-life care. The following section seeks to explore the impact of intersectional aspects of racism and cultural ignorance for people who are Black or hold minority identities and who also use substances at, or near, the end of their lives.

Taking an intersectional approach

Intersectionality was a concept first introduced by Crenshaw (1989) who identified the multiple and intersecting forms of inequality which often work together, compound each other and are contextually affected by social, historical and political factors. This analytical framework can act as a lens through which we can look at the complexity of how discrimination works, how individuals experience it and how society responds to it. This shows how the multiple layers of discrimination (such as race, gender, caste, religion, culture, sexuality, class, disability, age and immigration status) intersect to increase disadvantage and inequality. In identifying how these different forms of discrimination and systems of power operate and impact on minoritized communities, we can look for ways to address these inequalities and promote a more equal society. A way of utilizing intersectionality to see the ways in which a person's life is impacted by the layers of discrimination is through using a case study approach.

Using intersectionality as a lens

The case study portrays a Muslim woman who has been ostracized by her family and community and is living in poverty, isolation and fear, a situation representative of the stigma surrounding women's alcohol use in many cultures (Valentine et al., 2010). Samira's lack of agency can be attributed to her gender, which can be a social division in life. From birth gender can impact the way woman are treated within society, and within both the family hierarchy and paternal system. Women

---

Box 11.1 Case study 1

Samira, a 68-year-old woman, was found collapsed in the street, and admitted to hospital with acute stomach pains, jaundice and a history of vomiting blood. She has not provided any details of next of kin, indicating that she does not want anyone contacted. She has limited English but identifies as being a Muslim, and from Pakistan. Medics confirm she has advanced cirrhosis of the liver caused by excessive alcohol consumption. Symptoms suggest that she is in the last weeks of life. Samira lives alone, in an area which is classed as deprived, and regularly faces racist abuse, which has got worse over recent years. She is fearful of crime, of personal physical violence, both when she goes out and when she is in her home. Because of this she only goes out when it is absolutely necessary and sleeps only when she blacks out from excess alcohol use. She has other long-term conditions, including depression, which are negatively impacting on her physical, mental and emotional wellbeing.

---

are frequently brought up with, and become accustomed to, male dominated power structures in their individual relationships as well as in the wider community (Napikoski and Lewis, 2019). The concepts of honour (*izzat*) and shame (*sharam*) are often apparent in such family dynamics, and used to control female behaviour (Jafri, 2009), with values passed on through generations (Peart, 2012). Such patriarchal values can be embedded in the traditions of closed communities, and as such may mean that female family members adopt a subservient role to men. They may not be permitted to exercise autonomy in decision making, or contact outside help (Sultana, 2011), factors that increase women's vulnerability and potential isolation (Vigil, 2011). In the case study, Samira had not had access to education, and consequently has no literacy or language skills. This is reflective of evidence showing that over 500 million females across the world have no literacy skills (UNESCO, 2016). In the UK 16.4% of the population have low literacy levels (National Literacy Trust, 2021) and 1.6% of the population (863,000 people) have limited or no ability to speak English of whom two thirds are female (Gov. UK, 2020). Literacy issues present fundamental challenges to accessing information, services, and support (Memon et al., 2016). There is also heightened vulnerability for women who have entered the country on a spousal visa: compounding their dependence and lack of autonomy (Styles, 2014). Certainly, an insecure immigration status can render women powerless, fearing that contact with professional services may lead to deportation (Bhuyan, 2008). In the case study, this may have prevented Samira from accessing healthcare sooner. Although women's immigration status can be remedied within two years of immigration, Roy (2008) asserts that many husbands intentionally do not secure the legal status of their wives. Furthermore, the silence which is imposed upon these women makes them susceptible to abuse, manipulation and isolation (Siddiqui, 2018). Additionally, information and guidance for families is often received through community and religious leaders who will be influential in individual's access to support (Bayliss et al., 2014). The case study shows how Samira's life has been oppressed on many levels, and how she has covered up her alcohol use, resulting in her severe social isolation. She has not engaged with health or social care services which could have given her treatment options, instead she presented to health services in a crisis situation. The case study draws attention to how Selina's alcohol use and absence of palliative care has been affected directly by racism. Past discriminatory treatment by healthcare staff accounts for her lack of trust for service providers, and her inability to sleep without becoming sedated by alcohol is due, in part, to the fear of the racist violence towards her.

Substance use among forced migrant populations is beginning to emerge as a global public health issue (Horyniak et al. 2016), although it remains an under researched area (Horyniak et al., 2016; Lo et al., 2017). The case study depicts how Mo was waiting for his status to be determined (which may take months, or years), and as an asylum seeker has limited rights, is restricted from working, claiming welfare benefit or moving out of temporary accommodation. This situation is true for over 258 million people who live as migrants, away from their country of birth (United Nations, 2017); 82.4 million people worldwide have been forcibly displaced by war or persecution and now live as refugees (UNHCR, 2021). Mo, like others, has been exposed to socioeconomic disadvantage (Leão et al., 2006), poor quality and/or multi occupancy housing which cause anxiety and distress. He also has little or no support network and is susceptible to mental health problems (Weissbecker et al., 2019). Racism, discrimination, violence and sexual abuse are commonly experienced by migrants, who are vulnerable to abuse and crime because of their insecure housing, unemployment, social isolation and lack of knowledge about accessing services and support (Langlois et al., 2016). Mo's story demonstrates how this vulnerability increased his likelihood of becoming involved in risky behaviours (Acartürk et al., 2011). Experiencing such trauma, leaving family behind and receiving so little support in the host country, again

---

Box 11.2 Case study 2

Mo is a 66-year-old man who was forced to migrate to England two years ago and remains in a hostel which is over-crowded and unsanitary. He is awaiting an outcome for his application to remain in the UK. Mo has experienced significant trauma throughout his life. He was forced to leave his family behind and endure a perilous journey to find himself in a hostile environment, where he cannot work, claim benefits or access healthcare. He has no knowledge of how health, employment or housing systems work, and because he cannot speak English, he receives information from other refugees and refugee agency officials. Mo started using illicit substances and alcohol to cope with his

predisposes migrants to alcohol and drug use (Lemmens et al., 2017). The case study also shows how Mo's lack of knowledge of services and fear of deportation prevented engagement with any healthcare provision (Fountain et al., 2004). Evidence shows that migrants experience more symptoms of depression (Missinne and Bracke, 2012) and stress-induced mental illness (Laban et al., 2007). For younger migrants, risky behaviour is often associated with their desire to fit in to the dominant culture. Acculturation describes this process of cultural, social and psychological change which occurs when individuals try to adapt to the dominant culture of the society where they are living, and often involves balancing their culture of origin and the prevailing culture. Evidence suggests that acculturation is related to drug use as individuals are introduced to unfamiliar norms and values amidst a desire to fit in (Abbot and Chase, 2008).

Summary

There are several gaps in the literature relating to alcohol use in certain marginalized groups and communities (Gleeson et al., 2019). At the same time, it is difficult to assess the true nature of substance use in people identifying as being from minoritized communities due to the stigma and religious/cultural prohibition, creating secrecy and silence. However, what is very evident is the structural inequalities and discrimination which face minoritized communities, increasing the risk of poor health and deprivation related behaviours as well as a mistrust in statutory services.

There appears to be issues which are generic to both palliative care and substance use services, with both areas indicating a gap between service use and service need and a disparity in representation (Bayley and Hurcombe, 2011; CQC, 2016; Gleeson et al., 2019). There is also an identified need to provide culturally appropriate services, which are sensitive to religious differences and needs to encourage access to services (Calanzani et al., 2013; Muslim Council of Britain, 2019). In the UK, General Practitioners (GPs) and primary care services provide the gateway to key services, although research suggests that those from minoritized backgrounds have had poor experiences engaging with GPs (Markham et al., 2014; CQC, 2016). In a report by Herring et al. (2019) it was found that referrals to alcohol and drug use services were not routinely followed up if patients failed to attend, while individuals with insecure immigration status or no recourse to public funds are not entitled to access services at all. Findings from a retrospective service evaluation (Chidiac et al., 2020) set in a UK general hospital during the COVID-19 pandemic found that patients from Black and minoritized backgrounds, especially women, were referred later to palliative care than White patients, consequently receiving suboptimal care. No studies were found explicitly looking at end-of-life care for people using substances from Black and minoritized backgrounds.

Implications for policy and practice

- Insufficient and inappropriate service provision represents the main structural and cultural barrier to those requiring support and treatment. Commissioners and policy makers need to better understand the gaps in provision and make services more inclusive.

- UK drug policies adversely affect Black and marginalized communities. Policy makers need to address the legislation to prevent further harm to vulnerable societal groups.
- To increase awareness among Black and minoritized communities of the whole range of community palliative services they could access, with information demonstrating how access to such services would not contravene religious beliefs. This will involve greater partnership working with faith leaders and community groups.
- Cultural competency is the process of developing skills to increase engagement with different cultures. It could be enhanced by providing mandatory training to frontline staff – with services developing religious literacy around the understanding of faiths and use of appropriate language.
- It is vital that refugees entering the host country are given information about PTSD and mental health conditions, alongside service provision, as research indicates that this is an area which often remains unaddressed (Jozaghi et al., 2016).
- Muslim leaders have highlighted the need to counter existing stigma around death and dying and increase the community's awareness of available services (Muslim Council of Britain, 2019). This work needs supporting and disseminating.

Concluding remarks

This chapter has highlighted the generic barriers for Black and minoritized communities accessing all healthcare services such as difficulty navigating services, false stereotyping, discrimination, lack of knowledge of services, lack of interpreters and lack of cultural or religious competency. We would contend that all of these factors can and should be addressed by service providers, to offer inclusive services to the most vulnerable people in society. There is also a likelihood that the UK will see a growth in substance use problems among second-generation minoritized communities as individuals try to adapt to the dominant culture of UK society. Such acculturation may potentially increase access to services as people learn how to navigate systems and receive education about substance use and treatments available.

References

Abbot, P. and Chase, D.M. (2008) 'Culture and substance abuse: Impact of culture affects approach to treatment.' *Psychiatric Times*, 25(1) pp. 43–43. GALE|A180317139

Aboul-Enein, B.H. (2016) 'Health-promoting verses as mentioned in the Holy Quran.' *Journal of Religion and Health*, 55(3) pp. 821–829. DOI: 10.1007/s10943-014-9857-8

Acartürk, C.Z., Nierkens, V., Agyemang, C. and Stronks, K. (2011) 'Depressive symptoms and smoking among young Turkish and Moroccan ethnic minority groups in the

Netherlands: a cross-sectional study.' *Substance Abuse Treatment Prevention and Policy,* 6(5). DOI: 10.1186/1747-597X-6-5

Aldridge, M.D. and Bradley, E.H. (2017) 'Epidemiology and patterns of care at the end of life: rising complexity, shifts in care patterns and sites of death.' *Health Affairs,* 36(7) pp. 1175–1183. DOI: 10.1377/hlthaff.2017.0182

Alexander, M. (2012) *The New Jim Crow: Mass Incarceration in the Age of Color Blindness.* New York: The New Press. ISBN: 978-1-62097-193-2.

Ali-Northcott, L. (2013) Substance abuse. *In* Ahmed, S. and Amer M.M. (eds.) *Counselling Muslims: Handbook of Mental Health Issues and Interventions.* Routledge, pp. 375–402. DOI: 10.3998/jmmh.10381607.0006.206

Askew, R. and Salinas, M. (2019) 'Status, stigma and stereotype: How drug takers and drug suppliers avoid negative labelling by virtue of their 'conventional' and 'law-abiding' lives.' *Criminology & Criminal Justice,* 19(3) pp. 311–327. DOI: 10.1177/1748895818762558

Bayley, M. and Hurcombe, R. (2011) 'Drinking patterns and alcohol service provision for different ethnic groups in the UK: a review of the literature.' *Ethnicity and Inequalities in Health and Social Care,* 3(4) pp. 6–17. DOI: 10.5042/eihsc.2011.0073

Bayliss, K., Riste, L., Fisher, L., Wearden, A., Peters, S., Lovell, K. and Chew-Graham, C. (2014) 'Diagnosis and management of chronic fatigue syndrome/myalgic encephalitis in black and minority ethnic people: a qualitative study.' *Primary Health Care Research and Development,* 15(2) pp. 143–155. DOI: 10.1017/S1463423613000145

Bhopal, R.S. (2014) *Migration, Ethnicity, Race, and Health in Multicultural Societies.* Oxford University Press. DOI: 10.1093/med/9780199667864.001.0001

Bhuyan, R. (2008) 'The production of the battered immigrant in public policy and domestic violence advocacy.' 23(2) pp. 153–170. DOI: 10.1177/0886260507308317

Black, C. (2020) *Review of Drugs - Evidence Relating to Drug Use, Supply and Effects, Including Current Trends and Future Risks.* Retrieved from: https://assets.publishing.service. gov.uk/government/uploads/system/uploads/attachment_data/file/882953/Review_of_ Drugs_Evidence_Pack.pdf [Accessed 10th March 2021].

Cain, C. L., Surbone, A., Elk, R. and Kagawa-Singer, M. (2018) 'Culture and palliative care: preferences, communication, meaning, and mutual decision making.' *Journal of Pain and Symptom Management,* 55(5) pp. 1408–1419. DOI: 10.1016/j.jpainsymman.2018.01.007

Calanzani, N., Higginson, I.J. and Gomes, B. (2013) *Current and Future Needs for Hospice Care: An Evidence-Based Report.* London: Commission into the Future of Hospice care. Retrieved from: https://www.basw.co.uk/system/files/resources/basw_103716-5_0. pdf [Accessed 5th October 2021].

Caldwell, T.M., Rodgers, B., Clark, C., Jefferis, B.J.M.H., Stansfeld, S.A. and Power, C. (2008) 'Lifecourse socioeconomic predictors of midlife drinking patterns, problems and abstention: findings from the 1958 British Birth Cohort Study.' *Drug and Alcohol Dependence,* 95(3) pp. 269–278. DOI: 10.1016/j.drugalcdep.2008.01.014

Care Quality Commission. (2016) *A different ending: Addressing inequalities in end of life care.* Newcastle upon Tyne: CQC. Retrieved from: https://www.cqc.org.uk/sites/default/ files/20160505%20CQC_EOLC_OVERVIEW_FINAL_3.pdf [Accessed 9th September 2021].

Casetta, B., Videla, A. J., Bardach, A., Morello, P., Soto, N., Lee, K., Camacho, P.A., Moquillaza, R.V.H. and Ciapponi, A. (2017) 'Association between cigarette smoking prevalence and income level: a systematic review and meta-analysis.' *Nicotine & Tobacco Research,* 19(12) pp. 1401–1407. DOI: 10.1093/ntr/ntw266

Chidiac, C., Feuer, D., Flatley, M., Rodgerson, A., Grayson, K. and Preston, N. (2020) 'The need for early referral to palliative care especially for Black, Asian and minority ethnic groups in a COVID-19 pandemic: findings from a service evaluation.' *Palliative Medicine*, 34(9) pp. 1241–1248. DOI: 10.1177/0269216320946688

Crenshaw, K. (1989) Demarginalizing the intersection of race and sex: A black feminist critique of antidiscrimination doctrine, feminist theory and antiracist politics. *University of Chicago Legal Forum*: Article 8.139. Retrieved from: http://chicagounbound.uchicago.edu/uclf/vol1989/iss1/8 [Accessed 14th September 2021].

Dixon, J., King, D., Matosevic, T., Clark, M. and Knapp, M. (2018) *Equity in the Provision of Palliative Care in the UK: Review of Evidence*. Personal Social Services Research Unit: London School of Economics. 2015. Retrieved from: www.mariecurie.org.uk/globalassets/media/documents/policy/campaigns/equity-palliative-care-uk-report-full-lse.pdf [Accessed 18th March, 2021].

Duffy, S. (2012) *A Fair Society: How the Cuts Target Disabled People*. Sheffield: The Centre for Welfare Reform, on behalf of the Campaign for a Fair Society. Retrieved from: http://www.centreforwelfarereform.org/library/type/pdfs/a-fair-society1.html. [Accessed 23rd March 2021].

Fountain, J., Khurana, J. and Underwood, S. (2004) *Barriers to Drug Service Access by Minority Ethnic Populations in the European Union and How They Can Begin to be Dismantled*. Retrieved from: http://www.drugtext.org/Minorities/barriers-to-drugservice-access-by-minorityethnic-populations-in-the-european-union-and-how-they-canbegin-to-bedismantled.html [Accessed 16th March 2021].

Galvani, S., Manders, G., Wadd, S. and Chaudhry, S. (2013) *Developing a Community Alcohol Support Package: An Exploration with a Punjabi Sikh Community*. Retrieved from: https://uobrep.openrepository.com/bitstream/handle/10547/603551/CASP-Final-Report-December-2013.pdf?sequence=2 [Accessed 8th June 2021].

Gleeson, H., Herring, R. and Bayley, M. (2020) 'Exploring gendered differences among polish migrants in the UK in problematic drinking and pathways into and through alcohol treatment.' *Journal of Ethnicity in Substance Abuse*, 1–21. DOI: 10.1080/15332640.2020.1836697

Gleeson, H., Thom, B., Bayley, M. and McQuarrie T. (2019) *Rapid Evidence Review: Drinking Problems and Interventions in Black and Minority Ethnic Communities*. Retrieved from: https://core.ac.uk/download/pdf/328319220.pdf [Accessed 23rd March 2021].

GOV.UK. (2020) *English Language Skills*. https://www.ethnicity-facts-figures.service.gov.uk/uk-population-by-ethnicity/demographics/english-language-skills/latest#main-facts-and-figures [Accessed 25th March 2021].

Harries, B., Harris, S., Hall, N. and Cotterell, N. (2019) 'Lessons for practice and policy. Older BAME people's experiences of health and social care in Greater Manchester.' Retrieved from: http://www.oldham-council.co.uk/jsna/wp-content/uploads/2018/11/BAME-peoples-experiences-of-health-and-social-care.pdf [Accessed 25th March 2021].

Hart, B., Sainsbury, P. and Short, S. (1998) '"Whose dying?" A sociological critique of the good death.' *Mortality*, 3(1) pp. 65–77. DOI: 10.1080/713685884

Herring, R., Gleeson, H. and Bayley, M. (2019) *Exploring pathways through and beyond alcohol treatment among Polish women and men in a London Borough*. Alcohol Change UK, Retrieved from: https://s3.eu-west-2.amazonaws.com/files.alcoholchange.org.uk/documents/Exploring-alcohol-treatment-among-Polish-adults_Final-Report.pdf [Accessed 8th November 2021].

Home Office. (2020) *Police Powers and Procedures, England and Wales, Year Ending 31 March 2020 – Second Edition*. Retrieved from: https://assets.publishing.service.gov.uk/government/uploads/system/uploads/attachment_data/file/935355/police-powers-procedures-mar20-hosb3120.pdf [Accessed 8th November, 2021].

Horyniak, D., Melo, J.S., Farrell, R.M., Ojeda, V.D. and Strathdee, S.A. (2016) 'Epidemiology of substance use among forced migrants: A global systematic review.' *PLoS One, 11*(7) p. e0159134. DOI: 10.1371/journal.pone.0159134

Howarth, G. (2007) *Death and Dying: A Sociological Introduction.* Cambridge: Polity Press. ISBN: 978-0-745–62533-1

Hurcombe, R., Bayley, M. and Goodman, A. (2010) *Ethnicity and Alcohol: A Review of the UK Literature.* Project Report. Joseph Rowntree Foundation, York. Retrieved from: https://eprints.mdx.ac.uk/7951/1/Hurcombe-ethnicity-alcohol-literature-review-full_0.pdf [Accessed 29th March 2021].

Jafri, A.H. (2009) *Honour Killing: Dilemma, Ritual and Understanding.* Oxford: Oxford University Press. ISBN: 9780195476316.

Jones, L., McCoy, E., Bates, G., Bellis, M.A. and Sumnall, H.R. (2015) *Understanding the Alcohol Harm Paradox in Order to Focus the Development of Interventions.* Alcohol Research UK. Retrieved from: https://s3.eu-west-2.amazonaws.com/files.alcoholchange.org.uk/documents/FinalReport_0122.pdf?mtime=20181109150106 [Accessed 10th March 2021].

Jozaghi, E., Asadullah, M. and Dahya, A. (2016) 'The role of Muslim faith-based programs in transforming the lives of people suffering with mental health and addiction problems.' *Journal of Substance Use, 21*(6) pp. 587–593. DOI: 10.3109/14659891.2015.1112851

Kim, S., Hahm, K.H., Park, H.W., Kang, H.H. and Sohn, M. (2010) 'A Korean perspective on developing global policy for advance directives.' *Bioethics, 24*, pp. 113–117. DOI: 10.1111/j.1467-8519.2009.01787.x

King's Fund. (2020) *Ethnic Minority Deaths and Covid-19: What Are We To Do?* Retrieved from: https://www.kingsfund.org.uk/blog/2020/04/ethnic-minority-deaths-covid-19 [Accessed 12th September 2021].

King's Fund. (2021) *The Health of People from Ethnic Minority Groups in England.* Retrieved from: https://www.kingsfund.org.uk/publications/health-people-ethnic-minority-groups-england#conclusion [Accessed 14th October 2021].

Koffman, J. (2018) *Dementia and End of Life Care for Black, Asian and Minority Ethnic Communities.* Retrieved from: https://raceequalityfoundation.org.uk/wp-content/uploads/2018/07/REF-Better-Health-451-1.pdf [Accessed 22nd March 2021].

Laban, C.J., Gernaat, H.B., Komproe, I.H. and De Jong, J.T. (2007) 'Prevalence and predictors of health service use among Iraqi asylum seekers in the Netherlands.' *Social Psychiatry and Psychiatric Epidemiology, 42*(10) pp. 837–844. DOI: 10.1007/s00127-007-0240-x

Langlois, E.V., Haines, A., Tomson, G. and Ghaffar, A. (2016) 'Refugees: towards better access to health-care services.' *The Lancet, 387*(10016) pp. 319–321. DOI: 10.1016/S0140–6736(16)00101-X

Leão, T.S., Johansson, L.M. and Sundquist, K. (2006) 'Hospitalization due to alcohol and drug abuse in first- and second-generation immigrants: a follow-up study in Sweden.' *Substance Use and Misuse, 41*(3) pp. 283–296. DOI: 10.1080/10826080500409100

Lemmens, P., Dupont, H. and Roosen, I. (2017) *Migrants, Asylum Seekers and Refugees: an Overview of the Literature Relating to Drug Use and Access to Services.* Background paper commissioned by the EMCDDA. Background paper commissioned by the EMCDDA for Health and social responses to drug problems: a European guide, EMCDDA, Lisbon. Retrieved from: https://www.emcdda.europa.eu/system/files/attachments/6341/EuropeanResponsesGuide2017_BackgroundPaper-Migrants-Asylum-seekers-Refugees-Drug-use.pdf [Accessed 12th September 2021].

Lo, J., Patel, P., Shultz, J. M., Ezard, N. and Roberts, B. (2017) 'A systematic review on harmful alcohol use among civilian populations affected by armed conflict in low- and middle-income countries.' *Substance Use & Misuse, 52*(11) pp. 1494–1510. DOI: 10.1080/10826084.2017.1289411

Maciagowska, K.E. and Hanley, T. (2017) 'What is known about mental health needs of the post-European Union accession Polish immigrants in the UK? A systematic review.' *International Journal of Culture and Mental Health, 11*(2) pp. 220–235. DOI: 10.1080/17542863.2017.1358755

Mallik, S., Starrels, J.L., Shannon, C., Edwards, K. and Nahvi, S. (2021) '"An undercover problem in the Muslim community": A qualitative study of imams' perspectives on substance use.' *Journal of Substance Abuse Treatment, 123* p. 108224. DOI: 10.1016/j.jsat.2020.108224

Manickam, M.A., Abdul Mutalip, M.H.B., Hamid, H.A.B.A., Bt Kamaruddin, R. and Sabtu, M.Y.B. (2014) 'Prevalence, comorbidities, and cofactors associated with alcohol consumption among school-going adolescents in Malaysia.' *Asia Pacific Journal of Public Health, 26*(5_suppl) pp. 91S–99S. DOI: 10.1177/1010539514542194

Markham, S., Islam, Z. and Faull, C. (2014) 'I never knew that! Why do people from Black and Asian Minority Ethnic groups in Leicester access hospice services less than other groups? A discussion with community groups.' *Diversity & Equality in Health & Care, 11.* Retrieved from: https://loros.co.uk/assets/i_never_knew_that_markham_islam_and_faull_2014.pdf [Accessed 15th September 2021].

Marmot, M. (2010) *Fair Society, Healthy Lives: Strategic Review of Health Inequalities in England Post 2010.* London: University College London. Retrieved from: https://www.instituteofhealthequity.org/resources-reports/fair-society-healthy-lives-the-marmot-review/fair-society-healthy-lives-full-report-pdf.pdf [Accessed 12th October 2021].

Marmot, M. (2020) 'Health equity in England: the Marmot review 10 years on.' *British Medical Journal, 368.* DOI: 10.1136/bmj.m693

Mauseth, K.B., Skalisky, J., Clark, N.E. and Kaffer, R. (2016) 'Substance use in Muslim culture: social and generational changes in acceptance and practice in Jordan.' *Journal of Religion and Health, 55*(4) pp. 1312–1325. DOI: 10.1007/s10943-015-0064-z

Meier, D. E., Isaacs, S. L. and Hughes, R. (Eds.). (2011) *Palliative Care: Transforming the Care of Serious Illness* (Vol. 33). John Wiley & Sons. ISBN: 978-0-470-52717-7

Memon, A., Taylor, K., Mohebati, L.M., Sundin, J., Cooper, M., Scanlon, T. and de Visser, R. (2016) 'Perceived barriers to accessing mental health services among Black and minority ethnic (BME) communities: a qualitative study in Southeast England.' *BMJ Open, 6*(11). DOI: http://dx.doi.org/10.1136/bmjopen-2016-012337

Missinne, S. and Bracke, P. (2012) 'Depressive symptoms among immigrants and ethnic minorities: a population based study in 23 European countries.' *Social Psychiatry and Psychiatric Epidemiology, 47*(1) pp. 97–109. DOI: 10.1007/s00127-010-0321-0

Motune, V. (2011) *Secret Lives.* Alcohol: BME Services. 22–23. Retrieved from: http://www.drinkanddrugsnews.com/magazine/440e6d1991bb4dc689483762aa39abf   5.pdf [Accessed 15th September 2021].

Muslim Council of Britain. (2019) *Elderly & End of Life Care for Muslims in the UK.* Retrieved from: https://mcb.org.uk/wp-content/uploads/2019/08/MCB_ELC_Web.pdf [Accessed 25th March 2021].

Napikoski, L. and Lewis, J.J. (2019) *Oppression and Women's History.* Retrieved from: www.thoughtco.com [Accessed 15th September 2021].

National Literacy Trust. (2021) *Adult Literacy.* Retrieved from: https://literacytrust.org.uk/parents-and-families/adult-literacy/ [Accessed 25th March 2021].

Office for National Statistics. (2020) *Population of the UK by Country of Birth and Nationality: 2020.* Retrieved from: https://www.ons.gov.uk/peoplepopulationand

community/populationandmigration/internationalmigration/bulletins/ukpopulationby
countryofbirthandnationality/2020 [Accessed 8th November 2021].

Oliffe, J.L., Grewal, S., Bottorff, J.L., Dhesi, J., Bindy, H., Kang, K. and Hislop, T.G. (2010) 'Masculinities, diet and senior Punjabi Sikh immigrant men: Food for western thought?' *Sociology of Health and Illness*, 32 pp. 761–776. Palliative Care; 19 pp. 133–139. DOI: 10.1111/j.1467-9566.2010.01252.x

Parkes, C.M., Laungani, P. and Young, W. (eds.) (2015) *Death and Bereavement across Cultures*. Routledge. ISBN: 9780415522366

Peart, K.K. (2012) 'Izzat and the gaze of culture.' *Crossings: Journal of Migration and Culture*, 3(1) pp. 53–70. DOI: 10.1386/cjmc.3.1.53_1

Public Health England. (2016) *The Public Health Burden of Alcohol and the Effectiveness and Cost-Effectiveness of Alcohol Control Policies: An Evidence Review*. Retrieved from: https://assets.publishing.service.gov.uk/government/uploads/system/uploads/attachment_data/file/733108/alcohol_public_health_burden_evidence_review_update_2018.pdf [Accessed 10th March, 2021].

Public Health England. (2020) *Adult Substance Misuse Treatment Statistics 2019 to 2020: Report*. Retrieved from: https://www.gov.uk/government/statistics/substance-misuse-treatment-for-adults-statistics-2019-to-2020/adult-substance-misuse-treatment-statistics-2019-to-2020-report [Accessed 8th November 2021].

Richards, N. and Krawczyk, M. (2021) 'What is the cultural value of dying in an era of assisted dying?' *Medical Humanities*, 47(1) pp. 61–67. DOI: 10.1136/medhum-2018–011621

Roy, S. (2008) 'No recourse – No duty to care? Experiences of BAMER women and children affected by domestic violence and insecure immigration status in the UK.' London: Imkaan. Retrieved from: https://static1.squarespace.com/static/5f7d9f4addc689717e6ea200/t/61e6a77f9b3bf9708d007261/1642506112688/2008+_+Imkaan+_+No+Recourse+-+No+Duty+to+Care.pdf [Accessed 8th November 2021].

Siddiqui, H. (2018) 'Counting the cost: BME women and gender-based violence in the UK.' *IPPR Progressive Review*, 24(4) pp. 361–368. https://doi.org/10.1111/newe.12076

Smith, A.K., Thai, J.N., Bakitas, M.A., Meier, D.E., Spragens, L.H., Temel, J.S., Weissman, D.E. and Rabow, M.W. (2013). The diverse landscape of palliative care clinics. *Journal of Palliative Medicine*, 16(6) pp. 661–668. DOI: 10.1089/jpm.2012.0469

Social Metrics Commission. (2020) *Measuring Poverty*. Retrieved from: https://socialmetricscommission.org.uk/wp-content/uploads/2020/06/Measuring-Poverty-2020-Web.pdf [Accessed 15th September 2021].

Styles, T.S. (2014) *An Exploration of the Specialised Service Provision for BME Women who have Experienced Domestic Violence with Reference to Three Support Providers in the North West of England* (Doctoral dissertation, University of Central Lancashire). Retrieved from:http://clok.uclan.ac.uk/10758/2/Styles%20Tara%20Final%20eThesis%20%28Master%20Copy%29.pdf [Accessed 1st September 2021].

Sultana, A. (2011) 'Patriarchy and women s subordination: a theoretical analysis.' *Arts Faculty Journal*, 4 pp. 1–18. DOI: https://doi.org/10.3329/afj.v4i0.12929

Taak, K., Brown, J. and Perski, O. (2021) 'Exploring views on alcohol consumption and digital support for alcohol reduction in UK-based Punjabi-Sikh men: a think aloud and interview study.' *Drug and Alcohol Review*, 40(2) pp. 231–238. DOI: 10.1111/dar.13172

Thickett, A. and Bayley, M. (2013) *A Feasibility Study to Explore Alcohol Service Engagement among Polish Street Drinkers in a London Borough: Final report*. Alcohol Research UK, Drug and Alcohol Research Centre, Middlesex University. Retrieved from https://s3.eu-west-2.amazonaws.com/files.alcoholchange.org.uk/documents/FinalReport_0107.pdf [Accessed 15th September 2021].

Thom, B., Lloyd, C., Hurcombe, R., Bayley, M., Stone, K., Thickett, A. and Watts, B. (2010) *Black and Minority Ethnic Groups and Alcohol: A Scoping and Consultation Study.* London: Department of Health. Retrieved from: http://www.alcohollearningcentre.org. uk/_library/BME_report_final_draft_30_ July_2010_v4.pdf [Accessed 1st March 2021].

UK Drug Policy Commission. (2010) *The Impact of Drugs on Different Minority Groups: A Review Of The UK Literature.* Retrieved from: https://www.ukdpc.org.uk/wpcontent/ uploads/Evidence%20review%20-%20The%20impact%20of%20drugs%20on%20different%20minority%20groups_%20ethnic%20groups.pdf [Accessed 1st March 2021].

UK Parliament. (2020) *House of Commons Library: Ethnic Diversity in Politics and Public Life.* Retrieved from: https://commonslibrary.parliament.uk/research-briefings/sn01156/ [Accessed 8th March 2021].

UNESCO. (2016) *Global Education Monitoring Report 2016: Gender Review — Creating Sustainable Futures for All.* Retrieved from: https://en.unesco.org/gem-report/gender-reviews [Accessed 25th March 2021].

United Nations. (2017) *International Migration Report 2017: Highlights.* Retrieved from: https://www.un.org/en/development/desa/population/migration/publications/migration report/docs/MigrationReport2017_Highlights.pdf [Accessed 9th March 2021].

United Nations Human Rights Council. (UNHCR) (2021a) *Figures at a Glance.* Retrieved from: https://www.unhcr.org/figures-at-a-glance.html [Accessed 16th March 2021].

United Nations Human Rights Council. (2021b) *Arbitrary detention relating to drug policies: study of the working group on arbitrary detention.* Retrieved from: https://www.ohchr. org/Documents/Issues/Detention/Call/A_HRC_47_40_AdvanceEditedVersion.pdf [Accessed 8th March 2021].

Valentine, G., Holloway, S.L. and Jayne, M. (2010) 'Contemporary cultures of abstinence and the night time economy: Muslim attitudes towards alcohol and the implications for social cohesion.' *Environment and Planning A,* 42(1) pp. 8–22. DOI: 10.1068/a41303

Valentine, G., Sporton, D. and Nielsen, K.B. (2009) 'Identities and belonging: a study of Somali refugee and asylum seekers living in the UK and Denmark.' *Environment and Planning D: Society and Space,* 27(2) pp. 234–250. DOI: 10.1068/d3407

Vigil, S.F. (2011) *Giving Young Females a Voice: Perspectives of Somali Bantu Refugees Participating in a Wellness and Leadership Development Program.* Doctoral dissertation, University of Pittsburgh. Retrieved from: http://d-scholarship.pitt.edu/6746/1/StefanieVigil2011. pdf [Accessed 1st September 2021].

Weissbecker, I., Hanna, F., El Shazly, M., Gao, J. and Ventevogel, P. (2019) Integrative mental health and psychosocial support interventions for refugees in humanitarian crisis settings. *In* Wenzel, T. and Drožđek, B. (eds.) *An Uncertain Safety.* Cham: Springer, pp. 117–153. DOI: 10.1007/978-3-319-72914-5_6

Wicher, C.P. and Meeker, M.A. (2012) 'What influences African American end-of-life preferences.' *Journal of Health Care for the Poor and Underserved,* 23 pp. 28–58. DOI: 10.1353/hpu.2012.0027

Worster, B., Bell, D.K., Roy, V., Cunningham, A., LaNoue, M. and Parks, S. (2018) 'Race as a predictor of palliative care referral time, hospice utilization, and hospital length of stay: a retrospective noncomparative analysis.' *American Journal of Hospice and Palliative Medicine,* 35(1) pp. 110–116. DOI: 10.1177/1049909116686733

12 Unequal in life and death

Substance use, disadvantage and end-of-life care in prison

Marian Peacock and Mary Turner

Introduction

This chapter will consider the issues raised by the increase in what can be called 'anticipated' deaths in prisons in England and Wales, where palliative or end-of-life care may be applicable; it will also consider the wider context for this increase. This wider context raises a multiplicity of issues and questions as prison populations continue their steady rise, with particularly rapid growth in the older prisoner population, increasing health and social inequalities both inside and outside prisons and the changing pattern of these inequalities increasingly reflected in the prison population. Here we are focussing on the patterns of social and economic inequalities which intersect with, and underpin, other inequalities also well known in the prisons system such as ethnic, gender or religious discrimination.

The changes result in a picture of both disparate and intersecting inequalities within prisons, some of which are already presenting significant challenges to Her Majesty's Prison and Probation Service (HMPPS), and others that are indicative trends likely to raise challenges in the future if left unaddressed. These are:

- Patterns of inequality and disadvantage in prisons
- The disadvantaged body in prisons and the place of substance use
- Ageing and dying in prisons.

This chapter will examine these issues and will use two pen portraits to illustrate something of the breadth and complexity of the challenges faced. To ensure confidentiality, the pen portraits are not of specific individuals but rather are composites drawn from real-life experiences of people in prison and from our previous research (Turner and Peacock, 2017; Peacock et al., 2018; Turner et al., 2018). HMPPS has faced unprecedented challenges in recent decades, with Covid-19 adding further serious difficulties and widening existing inequalities, the consequences of which will only become fully clear over time. The pen portraits raise policy and practical challenges for prisons and illustrate suffering and a sharpening of existing disadvantage for the prisoners whose experiences they reflect.

DOI: 10.4324/9781003187882-15

Patterns of inequality and disadvantage in prisons

There is a long-standing history of prison populations having disproportionately high rates of ill health, deprivation and social and educational disadvantage (Prison Reform Trust, 2021). Prisoners typically have high rates of physical and mental ill health, substance use, learning difficulties, head injuries and a lack of literacy skills, as well as childhoods characterised by abuse and neglect (Fazel et al., 2016; Moynan et al., 2018; Hunter et al., 2021). It has been argued that there is a 'pipeline' from childhood experiences such as school exclusion, looked after status, childhood bereavement and suffering, to crime, substance use, being abused and/or abusing others and incarceration (Bowen et al., 2018; Novak, 2019). Demographically, prisoners are largely drawn from the most deprived areas of the United Kingdom (UK) and the patterns of ill health, suffering and deprivation mirror each other inside and outside prisons. The social and health composition of prisons does not reflect society as a whole, but does reflect social inequalities, in that the patterns are the same as those found in the most deprived populations.

The focus of this chapter is the prisons system in England and Wales (Scotland and Northern Ireland have different systems, making aggregating data or precise comparisons difficult), although arguably many of the patterns of deprivation and resultant incarceration are applicable in whole or in part to other populations. There are wide ranging inequalities both within prisons and within the disadvantaged and marginalised external populations from which prisoners disproportionately originate. Multiple, complex and intersecting patterns of inequality and disadvantage (for example, ethnicity) characterise both these populations but the complexity of these is outside the scope of this chapter. We will therefore focus on the economic and social inequalities which underpin and intersect with other inequalities.

The UK has the highest rate of imprisonment in Western Europe, with 140 prisoners per 100,000 of the population in England and Wales (compared with 100 in France and 61 in the Netherlands) (Walmsley, 2018), and this is projected to continue to rise over the coming years. There is little evidence of it being driven by crime rates, but rather by political decisions about sentence length and recall procedures, resulting in greater numbers of prisoners serving longer sentences. This is particularly the case amongst the older prisoner population. We will address some of the health and wellbeing issues in the older prisoner population when looking at ageing and dying below, but here it is worth noting that the increase in incarceration, primarily for historic sexual offences, in old age and for long sentences (which, although still relatively small in numbers reflects a growing trend) has had two impacts on patterns of health inequalities that may appear contradictory. On the one hand, there has been a significant increase in the numbers of the old and the 'oldest old' (Lee et al., 2018), who bring complex physical and mental health problems and serious disabilities associated with ageing. On the other hand, however, there is a subsection of this population who differ markedly from the economically and socially disadvantaged populations that make up the majority of prisoners. These are almost exclusively men who have had a greater degree of affluence and status prior to imprisonment, as illustrated in the pen portrait of Adrian (below). Some in this group do not bring the disadvantaged body of poverty and deprivation but rather a healthier body and more social challenges to prisons and prison officers. This latter increase is primarily due to convictions for 'historic' sexual abuse, resulting from greater awareness within the criminal justice system of the scale of childhood and adult sexual abuse, and a greater willingness to believe victims and survivors.

Patterns of deprivation in prisons reflect the patterns in the deprived areas from which prisoners disproportionately come. Drilling down into these patterns in more detail shows high rates of prescription of antidepressants and psychotropic drugs more widely, as well as high and rising rates of chronic pain, hand in hand with concerns around the rates of long-term prescribing of opioids. Life expectancy in deprived areas is low, and there is some evidence that this is now falling (Hiam et al., 2018). This trend is also mirrored in prison and is shown most starkly amongst homeless people, as incarceration disproportionately follows and precedes homelessness and substance use (Herbert et al., 2015; Aldridge et al., 2018). Frances Crook (Chief Executive of the Howard League for Penal Reform for 35 years), in an article in the Guardian, argues that prisons are 'black holes, into which society banishes those it deems problematic', and goes on to say: 'Prison is an unhealthy place. Most prisoners have come from poverty, addiction and social deprivation cemented by decades of failed social policy. Many arrive with long-term health problems, and in prison their health deteriorates further' (Crook, 2021). Addiction and its health consequences will now be considered.

The disadvantaged body in prisons and the place of substance use

Patterns of substance use outside prison are markedly impacted upon by social deprivation and, as would be expected, those coming into prison have higher rates of substance use than the population at large. There are three areas that need to be explored in thinking about substance use in prisons; first, what are the patterns of use as people come into prisons; second, what happens when people are incarcerated (does their drug use change and in what ways), and third, what are the patterns as people leave prison. These three areas raise policy and good governance challenges as well as questions about how prisons might respond more effectively.

A screening programme carried out in ten prisons in North West England in 2014 and 2015 found that 58% of prisoners on first reception to prison tested positive for substance use, with cannabis (25%), cocaine (25%) and heroin (17%) most commonly detected (Public Health England, 2017). There were also high levels of prescribed medications, in particular benzodiazepines, present in 22% of on-reception samples. These figures were based on testing data and are likely to be broadly reflective of patterns across England and Wales, but with some regional variations.

Once prisoners are incarcerated the patterns shift. There are two ways that the prevalence of substance use is measured in prisons; random drug tests and various self-report surveys have been undertaken to try to capture the wider experience of prisoners. Clearly these figures can only be indicative, but there is a substantial body of data, so they arguably have considerable validity. What these scores show is that there is a shift away from stimulant to sedative drugs, with cannabis being the most widely reported drug (used by 15% of prisoners) (Public Health England, 2017). The testing data shows a slightly different pattern with synthetic cannabinoid receptor antagonists (SCRAs), which were the only substances that increased during imprisonment. The picture is evolving as prisons struggle to manage this crisis, so accurate and up-to-date data may show changing patterns. This shift is empirically evidenced in drug-related deaths, with this being comparable to the broader population (Office of National Statistics, 2018). However, we are not focussing here on obvious drug-related deaths (for example, from homicide or suicide), but on the consequences of drug use over time, resulting in high rates of cancers and circulatory diseases which are the most common anticipated deaths in prisons, and are more likely to appear at an earlier age than in the non-substance using population both inside and outside prison.

In summary, this means that the substances being used change over the course of incarceration and release. For some, this means the acquisition of a habit they did not previously have, for others a change in the substance choice/use, and for some an end to or reduction in substance use. Similarly, on release these shifts raise varying risks of accidental overdose in those who attempt to return rapidly to pre-prison levels of consumption or new and potentially dangerous substance use habits.

Box 12.1 Pen portrait 1: Martin

Martin is a 65-year-old man who is serving the most recent of numerous custodial sentences. He was in care as a child and has had intermittent difficulties with alcohol throughout his life. He struggles with his feelings and mood, and many of his convictions are for impulsive violence when drunk, bitterly regretted when sober. He has numerous health problems, including chronic obstructive pulmonary disease, cardiovascular disease and liver disease, and is becoming increasingly frail.

The prison he is in has an Older Prisoner Unit (OPU), where Martin would have better access to health and social care, and where he would be safer. Although his growing frailty terrifies him and has already resulted in bullying and theft of his medication, Martin absolutely refuses to transfer to the OPU as it is 'on the VP side' of the prison. VP means vulnerable prisoner, but in prisons this is seen as synonymous with sex offenders because the majority of VPs have been imprisoned for sexual offences. VP is a highly stigmatised identity and one which non-VP prisoners dread and fear. Martin would prefer to suffer more where he is, rather than assume this 'spoiled identity' (Goffman, 2009).

Older prisoners have much lower rates of substance use than younger prisoners, but there are some indications that they have higher rates of problematic alcohol use prior to incarceration (Haesen et al., 2019), as exemplified in the pen portrait of Martin. Alcohol use is also strongly associated with a risk of premature death even when drinking cannot be continued in prison, as the most serious and life-limiting effects of heavy alcohol use are often only evident as people age. For other types of substance use there are two sets of issues that raise serious concern in prison; first, the falling numbers of prisoners able to access drug treatment programmes whilst incarcerated (O'Connor, 2018), and second, the burgeoning use of SCRAs (Kirby, 2016; Grace et al., 2020). This has been described as a 'natural experiment', where the consequences and outcomes may not be understood for decades. As well as the better-known effects of SCRAs such as collapse, stupor and, in a minority, death, the long-term effects on the brain and bodily organs over time suggest a potential 'epidemic' of dementia as these longer-term damages become apparent.

Ageing and dying in prison

The number of deaths from natural causes in prisons in England and Wales has been steadily increasing for several years, and the majority of these are in the older population. The experience of being in prison, particularly for a long period of time, is known to lead to premature ageing of about ten years, so that a prisoner aged 50 can expect to have an equivalent health status to someone aged 60 in the general population (Hayes et al., 2012). As Crook (2021) comments: 'While life expectancy and the quality of life for much of the country has advanced significantly in the past three decades, prisoners are considered "old" at 50'.

Because of the ageing effects of imprisonment, it is widely accepted that prisoners over the age of 50 should be classed as 'older' prisoners. At the time of writing, there are currently over 13,200 people aged over 50 in prison (17% of the prison population); 3,263 are in their 1960s and 1,693 are aged 70 or over (Prison Reform Trust, 2021). The prison population is projected to increase by over a quarter from 79,235 in September 2020 to 98,700 by September 2026 (Ministry of Justice, 2020), and the older prisoner population is expected to rise accordingly. The ageing prisoner population means that increasing numbers of people will face the end of their life behind bars; there were 174 natural cause deaths in prisons in the year to September 2020 (PRT, 2021), an increase of 40% in the last ten years.

There are several reasons for the ageing prisoner population. To begin with, the general population is ageing, and prisoners, like people outside prison, are living longer than in the past. The courts are now handing down more punitive sentences for crimes that in the past would have attracted a shorter sentence, and there are more stringent conditions attached to being given early release, meaning that more people breach these conditions and are returned to prison. Courts are also more willing to imprison old people; 92% of 80-year-olds in prison (currently 315 people) were sentenced when they were 70 or older (PRT, 2021). Older people in prison do not constitute one homogenous group; the Prison Reform Trust

---

Box 12.2 Pen portrait 2: Adrian

Adrian is an 87-year-old ex-vicar, imprisoned for the first time at the age of 85 for historic abuse of young clergy many years ago. Shortly after starting his sentence, he suffered a severe stroke, leaving him significantly physically incapacitated, with uncertain cognitive impacts and severely impaired speech. He spends almost all his time in his cell, as there are several short flights of stairs to other areas of the wing and to the outside which he is unable to climb. There is a lift that can accommodate a wheelchair on the longest flight, but this is almost always broken.

To evidence that he has reduced his risk of reoffending (a pre-requisite for parole), Adrian needs to complete several courses. However, his mobility difficulties and uncertain levels of comprehension and speech make this impossible.

(2021) identifies four different profiles of older prisoners: repeat offenders, grown old in prison, short-term first-time prisoners and long-term first-time prisoners. A high proportion of first-time prisoners, like Adrian, are sex offenders; 44% of men over 50 and 87% of men over 80 are in prison for sexual offences (PRT, 2021). Many older prisoners and all sex offenders are classed as 'Vulnerable Prisoners' (VPs) because they are vulnerable to intimidation by other prisoners, and they are housed completely separately from other prisoners for their own protection in VP units. As a convicted sex offender, Adrian was automatically housed in a VP unit. However, Martin has never been in a VP unit and, despite his increasing vulnerability because of his age and frailty, he is vehemently opposed to being housed with sex offenders because of the stigma attached, even though it would be easier for him to access the care he needs in a VP unit. Importantly, many of the 'middle old' and 'oldest old' (75–85 and 85 and over; Lee et al., 2018) are serving 'de facto' life sentences; even those given relatively short sentences might spend the rest of their lives in prison because of their age and limited life expectancy at imprisonment, even though the crime for which they are being punished does not carry a life sentence.

Older people in prison typically have multiple and complex health and social care needs, including dementia, chronic illness and pain, frailty and other long-term conditions; this is illustrated by both pen portraits. The majority of older people in prison (59%) report having a long-standing illness or disability, compared with 27% of younger people (PRT, 2021), but access to healthcare is often limited; most prisons do not provide in-patient care, and there is usually a long waiting list to see a GP in prison. A small number of prisons have created palliative care suites (larger cells with room for a hospital bed, hoist, etc.), but they are not available to most people dying in prison. Social care also presents challenges and, although some prisoners do receive help with activities of daily living, prison officers and fellow prisoners often have to be involved in providing care and support in the hours when the carers are not there. Most older prisoners take at least one prescription medication, and many take multiple medications (Turner et al., 2018), raising numerous issues around timely delivery, safety and security, bullying and intimidation. The mental health of older prisoners is often poor, with many reporting high levels of anxiety, fear of bullying and intimidation and pessimism about the future (Turner et al., 2018).

Many of those in prison for the first time in later life have been found to be suffering from 'entry shock', as a consequence of the 'truly catastrophic event' of being imprisoned (Crawley and Sparks, 2006; p. 68). Life as these older prisoners have known it has changed forever, and many experience anxiety, depression and distress when they start their sentence. The psychological trauma of entry shock is made worse by unfamiliarity with prison routines and regimes and a lack of information about expectations (Peacock et al., 2018). The prison environment (as illustrated by the pen portrait of Adrian) is not suitable for old, frail or dying people; prisons after all were not built to house this population. Prisoners often have to walk substantial distances to access healthcare departments, chaplaincy, work/activities or outside space, yet a survey of older prisoners found that a quarter of the 127 respondents could not walk more than 100 metres, and almost a fifth could not manage stairs without assistance (Turner et al., 2018). Equipment required by this population, such as wheelchairs, hoists, hospital beds, etc., simply do not fit in most prison cells.

To meet the needs of older people, a few prisons have started to develop specialist provision, such as designated older prisoner units. Few of these are purpose built and most utilise existing accommodation, usually on the ground floor, with variable adaptations to make them suitable for older or disabled people. Many of these seem to be repurposed VP accommodation, which may be a significant disincentive for non-VP prisoners who are very reluctant to be associated with the highly stigmatised VP identity. However, the provision of specialist older prisoner units is very 'ad hoc' and variable. The Prison Reform Trust reports that prison inspectors found that: 'Whilst some prisons offered good facilities and age-specific activities, others had no specific provision and little meaningful activity for those not in work – in some prisons inspectors found retired people in prison locked up for most of the day' (PRT, 2021; p. 29).

Reducing inequalities at the end of life

The Prison Reform Trust (2021) bluntly points out that in England and Wales: 'We choose to send people to prison for a long time… and it's growing' (p. 11). We are clearly also choosing to send older people to prison, sometimes for a long time, even when it is likely that they will die there, and this places enormous strain on HMPPS and those trying to provide appropriate and necessary care.

It is important to consider the purpose of prison; is it to punish people for crimes committed, keep the public safe from dangerous criminals, or rehabilitate offenders back into society? Prison can arguably serve some or all of these goals, but there is tremendous ambivalence both politically and within the population.

Despite the wealth of evidence that most prison sentences do little or nothing to reduce recidivism, prison is still positioned as a place where lessons are learnt. Imprisonment is often seen as a replacement for justice, with longer and longer sentences being understood as the only way of taking crime seriously or addressing the rights and needs of victims. Rates of UK imprisonment have risen over years where crime rates have largely fallen or stayed flat and, even when taking into account the important and long ignored rates of contemporary and historic sexual abuse and the consequent increase in imprisonment, there is little evidence that this 'works'.

HMPPS policy places great emphasis on rehabilitation, with their pledge to 'provide safe and supportive environments, where people work through the reasons that caused them to offend and prepare for a more positive future' (HMPPS, 2021). It is a common misconception that people go to prison for punishment, whereas they go to prison *as* punishment – a subtle but important distinction, the punishment being deprivation of liberty. They should not therefore be dealt additional punishment, for example, in the form of reduced access to healthcare; on the contrary, they should receive the same standard of healthcare as they would outside of prison. This is known as the principle of equivalence and is enshrined in international agreements such as the United Nations Standard Minimum Rules on the Treatment of Prisoners, also known as the 'Nelson Mandela Rules' (United Nations Office on Drugs and Crime, 2015). Rule 24 (page 8) states that: 'Prisoners should enjoy the same standards of health care that are available in the community, and should have access to necessary health-care services free of charge without discrimination on the grounds of their legal status'. The principle of equivalence is endorsed by the End of Life Care Strategy (Department of Health, 2008), which clearly states that all people approaching the end of life should be able to access high-quality care, regardless of who they are or where they might be.

Therefore, if as a society we want to continue to imprison old, frail and dying people, we need to ensure that prisons can provide not only safe and secure environments but also adequate and appropriate health and social care for those who need it. As noted above, one possible solution is to create older prisoner units, with specialist facilities and equipment and suitably trained staff, to accommodate and care for this vulnerable population appropriately. Such units have the potential to narrow inequalities, by providing equivalent care to that available outside prison. However, there is also the risk that they could widen inequalities, by not being available to all prisoners in this group. Another option is to release or not imprison those who are unlikely to pose any physical risk to society because of their ill health or frailty; they can either be released on temporary licence (ROTL) or granted early release on compassionate grounds (ERCG). However, ERCG is extremely rare, as stringent conditions have to be met and the whole process takes time, which means that some die in prison whilst waiting for their application to be considered.

Crucially, however, there are wider ethics and justice questions that must be addressed and a public conversation to be had about what justice looks like. What do victims feel is just? How might crime be reduced before it is committed rather than after the event? Whilst specialist end of life provision for older prisoners and more age friendly conditions have a role to play, the questions about how the UK incarcerates so many people and whether this constitutes justice have to be addressed before inequalities can narrow and something closer to justice can be achieved.

References

Aldridge, R.W., Story, A., Hwang, S.W., Nordentoft, M., Luchenski, S.A., Hartwell, G., Tweed, E.J., Lewer, D., Katikireddi, S.V. and Hayward, A.C. (2018) 'Morbidity and mortality in homeless individuals, prisoners, sex workers, and individuals with substance use disorders in high-income countries: a systematic review and meta-analysis.' *The Lancet*, 391(10117), pp. 241–250. DOI: 10.1016/S0140-6736(17)31869-X

Bowen, K., Jarrett, M., Stahl, D., Forrester, A. and Valmaggia, L. (2018) 'The relationship between exposure to adverse life events in childhood and adolescent years and subsequent adult psychopathology in 49,163 adult prisoners: A systematic review.' *Personality and Individual Differences*, 131, pp. 74–92. DOI: 10.1016/j.paid.2018.04.023

Crawley, E. and Sparks, R. (2006) 'Is there life after imprisonment? How elderly men talk about imprisonment and release.' *Criminology and Criminal Justice*, 6(1), pp. 63–82. DOI: 10.1177/1748895806060667

Crook, F. (2021) 'The reform of prisons has been my life's work, but they are still utterly broken.' Available from: https://www.theguardian.com/commentisfree/2021/aug/10/reform-prisons-utterly-broken?ref=refind [Accessed 5th November, 2021].

Department of Health. (2008) *End of Life Care Strategy: Promoting High Quality Care for all Adults at the End of Life*. Department of Health, London. Available from: https://assets.publishing.service.gov.uk/government/uploads/system/uploads/attachment_data/file/136431/End_of_life_strategy.pdf [Accessed 8th November 2021].

Fazel, S., Hayes, A.J., Bartellas, K., Clerici, M. and Trestman, R. (2016) 'Mental health of prisoners: prevalence, adverse outcomes, and interventions.' *The Lancet Psychiatry*, 3(9), pp. 871–881. DOI: 10.1016/S2215-0366(16)30142-0

Goffman, E. (2009) *Stigma: Notes on the Management of Spoiled Identity*. Simon and Schuster Inc; New York. DOI: 10.12691/ajmsm-8-3-3

Grace, S., Lloyd, C. and Perry, A. (2020) 'The spice trail: transitions in synthetic cannabis receptor agonists (SCRAs) use in English prisons and on release.' *Drugs: Education, Prevention and Policy*, 27(4), pp. 271–281. DOI: 10.1080/09687637.2019.1684878

Haesen, S., Merkt, H., Imber, A., Elger, B. and Wangmo, T. (2019) 'Substance use and other mental health disorders among older prisoners.' *International Journal of Law and Psychiatry*, 62, pp. 20–31. DOI: 10.1016/j.ijlp.2018.10.004

Hayes, A.J., Burns, A., Turnbull, P. and Shaw, J.J. (2012) 'The health and social needs of older male prisoners.' *International Journal of Geriatric Psychology*, 27(11), pp. 1152–1162. DOI: 10.1002/gps.3761

Herbert, C.W., Morenoff, J.D. and Harding, D.J. (2015) 'Homelessness and housing insecurity among former prisoners.' *RSF: The Russell Sage Foundation Journal of the Social Sciences*, 1(2), pp. 44–79. DOI: 10.7758/rsf.2015.1.2.04

Her Majesty's Prison and Probation Service. (2021). https://www.gov.uk/government/organisations/her-majestys-prison-and-probation-service/about [Accessed 10th September 2021].

Hiam, L., Harrison, D., McKee, M. and Dorling, D. (2018) 'Why is life expectancy in England and Wales 'stalling'?' *Journal of Epidemiology and Community Health*, 72(5), pp. 404–408. DOI: 10.1136/jech-2017-210401

Hunter, R.M., Anderson, R., Kirkpatrick, T., Lennox, C., Warren, F., Taylor, R.S., Shaw, J., Haddad, M., Stirzaker, A. and Maguire, M. (2021) 'Economic evaluation of a complex intervention (Engager) for prisoners with common mental health problems, near to and after release: a cost-utility and cost-consequences analysis.' *The European Journal of Health Economics*, 23, pp. 193–210. DOI: 10.1007/s10198-021-01360-7

Kirby, T. (2016) 'New psychoactive substances in prisons: high and getting higher.' *The Lancet Psychiatry*, 3(8), pp. 709–710. DOI: 10.1016/s2215-0366(16)30178-x

Lee, S.B., Oh, J.H., Park, J.H., Choi, S.P. and Wee, J.H. (2018) 'Differences in youngest-old, middle-old and oldest-old patients who visit the emergency department.' *Clinical and Experimental Emergency Medicine*, 5(4), pp. 249–255. DOI: 10.15441%2Fceem.17.261

Ministry of Justice. (2020) *Prison Population Projections 2020–2026, England and Wales*. Available from: https://assets.publishing.service.gov.uk/government/uploads/system/uploads/attachment_data/file/938571/Prison_Population_Projections_2020_to_2026.pdf [Accessed 9th August 2021].

Moynan, C.R. and McMillan, T.M. (2018) 'Prevalence of head injury and associated disability in prison populations: A systematic review.' *The Journal of Head Trauma Rehabilitation*, 33(4), pp. 275–282. DOI: 10.1097/HTR.0000000000000354

Novak, A. (2019) 'The school-to-prison pipeline: An examination of the association between suspension and justice system involvement.' *Criminal Justice and Behavior*, 46(8), pp. 1165–1180. DOI: 10.1177/0093854819846917

O'Connor, R. (2018) *Public Health Matters Blog: What We Learned About Alcohol and Drug Treatment in Prisons from the 2016–17 Statistics*. Public Health England; London. Available from: https://publichealthmatters.blog.gov.uk/2018/01/31/what-we-learned-about-alcohol-and-drug-treatment-in-prisons-from-the-2016-17-statistics/ [Accessed 9th September 2021].

Office for National Statistics. (2018) *Drug-related deaths and suicide in prison custody in England and Wales: 2008–2016*. Available from: https://www.ons.gov.uk/peoplepopulationandcommunity/birthsdeathsandmarriages/deaths/articles/drugrelateddeathsandsuicideinprisoncustodyinenglandandwales/2008to2016 [Accessed 9th September 2021].

Peacock, M., Turner, M. and Varey, S. (2018) '"We call it jail craft": the erosion of the protective discourses drawn on by prison officers dealing with ageing and dying prisoners in the neoliberal, carceral system.' *Sociology*, 52(6), pp. 1152–1168. DOI: 10.1177%2F0038038517695060

Prison Reform Trust. (2021) *Bromley Briefings Prison Factfile, Winter 2021*. Available from: http://www.prisonreformtrust.org.uk/Portals/0/Documents/Bromley%20Briefings/Winter%202021%20Factfile%20final.pdf [Accessed 6th August 2021].

Public Health England. (2017) *United Kingdom Drug Situation: Focal Point Annual Report 2017*. Public Health England, London. https://www.gov.uk/government/publications/united-kingdom-drug-situation-focal-point-annual-report [Accessed 6th August 2021].

Turner, M. and Peacock, M. (2017) 'Palliative care in UK prisons: practical and emotional challenges for custodial staff, healthcare professionals and fellow prisoners.' *Journal of Correctional Healthcare*, 23(1), pp. 56–65. DOI: 10.1177/1078345816684847

Turner, M., Peacock, M., Payne, S., Fletcher, A. and Froggatt, K. (2018) 'Ageing and dying in the contemporary neoliberal prison system: exploring the 'double burden' for older prisoners.' *Social Science and Medicine*, 212, pp. 161–167. DOI: 10.1016/j. socscimed.2018.07.009.

United Nations Office on Drugs and Crime. (2015) *The United Nations Standard Minimum Rules for the Treatment of Prisoners*. Available from: https://www.unodc.org/documents/-justice-and-prison-reform/Nelson_Mandela_Rules-E-ebook.pdf [Accessed 10th September 2021].

Walmsley, R. (2018) *World Prison Population List: Twelfth Edition*. Available from: https:// prisonstudies.org/sites/default/files/resources/downloads/wppl_12.pdf [Accessed 9th August 2021].

13 Reflections and recommendations

Multiple disadvantage, substance use and end-of-life care

Sarah Galvani, Sam Wright and Gary Witham

This book set out to present empirical and practice-based evidence of the challenges people face at, or near, the end of their lives, when they use substances. The evidence explored here suggests the current system of care is failing to reach, or consider, people who are marginalised in our communities through their substance use, health literacy, ethnicity, disability, mental ill health, homelessness, criminal justice involvement or sex work.

This is not just a UK concern. The World Health Organisation (WHO) reports a lack of access to palliative care for the 40 million people estimated to need it worldwide, most of them living in countries with low or middle incomes. It identified key barriers including a lack of understanding about palliative care among 'policy makers, health professionals and the public' as well as barriers stemming from cultural beliefs around death and dying, for example (WHO, 2020, online). It also stated there were incorrect assumptions that palliative care is for cancer patients only or for people who are at the very end of life. Of particular relevance here is WHO's identification of a key barrier being people's 'misconceptions that improving access to opioid analgesia will lead to increased substance abuse' (World Health Organisation, 2022, online).

In the UK palliative and end-of-life care policy has acknowledged the ongoing exclusionary nature of its services although not specifically relating to people using substances (Care Quality Commission, 2016; National End of Life Care Intelligence Network (NEoLCIN), 2018). While it has made recommendations to address these failings (National Palliative and End of Life Care Partnership (NPELCP, 2015), there has been little progress (NPELCP, 2021). Statistics for services show people with cancer still have a significantly better chance of accessing formal palliative or end-of-life care services than other life limiting illnesses such as stroke, heart failure and pulmonary disease (NEoLCIN, 2018). The data also suggest that people from particular socio-demographic backgrounds, including marginalised and previously excluded groups, may account for the 'unwarranted variation' in palliative and end-of-life care access (NEoLCIN, 2018). Unwarranted variation is defined as 'variation that cannot be explained on the basis of illness, medical evidence, or patient preference' (Wennberg, 2010 cited by NEoLCIN, 2018).

Substance use services fare little better. After a decade of decimation of substance use services through severe funding cuts (Roscoe et al., 2022), figures are

DOI: 10.4324/9781003187882-16

showing alcohol and drug-related deaths are at the highest since records began (ONS, 2021a, 2021b). There are also concerns about drug-related deaths worldwide (European Monitoring Centre for Drugs and Drug Addiction (EMCDDA), 2019), with high levels in North America. European data are largely unreliable due to lack of recording and under-reporting, however, Germany, Turkey and Sweden all report high levels of drug-induced deaths (EMCDDA, 2019).

In the UK, older age groups are now among those with the most substance-related morbidity and mortality (Office for Health Improvement and Disparities (OHID), 2022) as they take their use of substances into older age. The service system in the UK and worldwide appears unable to cope with the current growth in demand for services our ageing population brings, but also the need to diversify its offer and respond effectively to the complex and multi-layered needs with which people present.

Complex needs require complex responses

What is challenging for practice, policy and research, is developing a response that understands and addresses the multiple and layered nature of those needs. For practitioners, policy makers and researchers, single-focussed needs are far easier to address, categorise and explore. Multiple, compounded and complex needs create a far 'messier' picture resulting in responses that can be more difficult, more time consuming and more resource intensive. But we must engage with the 'messiness' and consider what immediate changes can be made while planning responses that may take longer to resource and achieve (Galvani and Wright, 2019). Only then will we be able to begin to address the health and social injustices that people face in accessing care.

Reflective policy at organisational, local and national level is essential to begin to address social and health inequalities for people using substances at, or near, the end of their lives, particularly for those with additional and intersecting needs (Galvani and Wright, 2019). Ahmed and Chesterton (Chapter 11), refer to people experiencing 'multiple layers of discrimination' that combine to 'increase disadvantage and inequality'. Witham and Galvani (Chapter 6) refer to the coalescing of discrimination and health inequalities, while Wright et al. (Chapter 2) refer to people feeling 'undeserving of end-of-life care'. This internal and external discrimination is a common theme in many of the chapters in this book. Wherever possible, the social and health inequalities people experience have been expressed through the voices of people who participated in the research, the practice upon which the chapters are based, or through composite case studies drawn from years of the authors' experience. Policy, practice and research need to consider whether minority needs are only minority because the dominant discourse drowns out minority voices. While they are treated as discrete groups they will remain a minority, whereas added together these marginalised groups make up a more substantial population. We need to actively seek out, and reach out, to marginalised groups and provide more accessible and equitable care.

What we learn in this text, is that this is a group of people who are not solely navigating access to one or two specialist systems from the margins of society but are balancing a range of health and social care needs and negotiating a range of systems with different rules, processes and expectations. This, at a time when they are unwell, both physically and in terms of their mental and emotional health. Add to this mix the internalisation of stigma that is often 'weaponised' (Wright et al., Chapter 2) by some professionals towards people they have stereotyped and dismissed, and a picture emerges of people having a mountain to climb to get the care they deserve.

This chapter will seek to outline policy and practice considerations that have been drawn from the chapters and evidence in this text, as well as wider literature. It will then propose a new systems level approach that takes account of the intersectional and compounded nature of the characteristics that combine to marginalise many people from palliative and end-of-life care.

Good policy practice

The need to improve access to palliative and end-of-life care services, within the UK, was documented in 2015 in a policy document outlining six main 'ambitions' for future care (National Palliative and End of Life Care Partnership, 2015). This clearly had limited effect as, in 2021, the partnership produced a further document stating that more needed to be done to 'break the cycle of reports asking for change' and reemphasising the six ambitions within a framework for local action:

1   each person is seen as an individual
2   each person gets fair access to care
3   maximising comfort and wellbeing
4   care is co-ordinated
5   all staff are prepared to care
6   each community is prepared to help.

On a larger geographical scale, Payne et al. (2019) conducted consultation with 36 experts from Europe, North America and Australia to determine priorities for integrated palliative care. As with the UK's 'ambitions', the resulting recommendations highlighted the need for adequate education and preparation on palliative care for health and social care professionals, as well as care coordination, and advocacy.

The lack of policy for working with people with multiple needs at the end of life and the negative impact it had on their care has been raised repeatedly in this book. Higgs (Chapter 8) highlighted how the lack of *policies for managing the use of illicit opioids* on inpatient wards meant that people were not going to be transparent about their substance use – indeed they would do what they could to stop people finding out. Good policy development would actively 'uncover' the hidden population and address their needs. Galvani et al. (Chapter 3) flagged the absence of *policies relating to pain and symptom management where someone was using substances* – a concern that was evidenced in the existing literature and the newer research on which the chapter is based. The fear of over- and under-prescribing and inadvertently leaving someone in pain or potentially killing them is an incredible burden for professionals to carry and needs a consistent response.

Webb (Chapter 7) called for policy that would *enable holistic models of care* that integrated people's 'beliefs and psychosocial and cultural norms' akin to the Oyster Care Model in Belgium. Oyster Care began with 'thinking outside the box' when the needs of specific groups of people with severe and enduring mental ill health were 'in danger of being forgotten' (Decorte et al., 2020). Instead of trying to restrict their behaviours and freedoms, a more creative approach was introduced whereby the person's behaviour was permitted (within some boundaries) and overseen by a range of caregivers. Examples suggested that in being less restrictive, the behaviours improved and more positive relationships were developed. The authors referred to it as an 'exoskeleton' or external skeleton around a person with four pillars of care comprising, physical, psychological, existential and social care. It served the purpose of reducing harm to the individual and those around them by releasing the pressure on the person to conform. This approach is worthy of consideration for the care of people being discussed in this text and overcomes the unrealistic (and unsuccessful) expectations placed on people using substances with multiple needs at or near the end of their lives. The Oyster Care approach seems to embody the reality of a harm reduction framework while placing the person's needs, not the system's needs, at its core. Galvani et al. (Chapter 3) also called for a *harm reduction framework* – common in substance use services – to be applied to end-of-life care approaches thereby allowing for creative care that can respond to the fluctuating needs of people with multiple needs including substance use at the end of their lives.

The call for more holistic approaches was also a conclusion in Chapter 4 in relation to support for family members and carers, and the need to consider their own use of substances and their own health concerns. Indeed, *family support initiatives and policies* were lacking in the wider literature and were highlighted as a gap in service provision. Overlooking family support is short-sighted and costly given they are the primary caregiver for people at, or near, the end of life. Supporting family or informal caregivers to support their relative or friend makes economic sense in a social and health care system that is struggling to find adequate resource.

A repeated message from the chapters was the need to *counter stigma and discrimination*. They called for policies that sought to address it or highlighted the lack of policies in place. In the first guidance of its kind, Galvani and Wright (2019) produced policy guidelines for addressing substance use among people at or near the end of their lives at organisational, local and national levels. The guidelines were grounded in the views of a large group of policy makers in the City of Liverpool, England. Countering stigma was at the top of the policy standards requested by the group. While there is often a disconnect between well-meaning policy and practice delivery, policy can provide the framework and support for changing practice. What it demonstrated was the amount of work there is still to do, but that not everything required expenditure and additional resources, for example, training exchanges across organisations, champion or lead liaison roles, or regular meetings with 'other' specialists.

Practitioner level good practice

While we await the operationalisation of good policy intentions at a systems level, we also need to reflect on what individual practitioners can do to effect positive immediate change.

Some actions could be affected at an individual practitioner level. Indeed, most of the good policy and practice documented (Galvani and Wright, 2019; Galvani et al., 2019) were triggered by committed and driven individuals within front-line substance use or palliative and end-of-life care services. As Wright et al. (Chapter 4) point out, professionals hold power that can be used for positive and creative good practice or to further marginalise people. Social and health care practitioners are constantly tasked with reflecting on practice and developing their professional knowledge. Far less comfortable is the task of self-critique and identifying internalised prejudice and stigma. Box 13.1 sets out some of the key individual practitioner responses that can facilitate better care of people using substances at, or near, the end of their lives.

Brien's chapter (Chapter 10) led us through a very personal experience of caring for someone and reflected her actions, rationale and questioning of it. Her experience demonstrated much good practice in terms of her resilience, tolerance and understanding of the extreme vulnerability that 'Jane' experienced. But it also demonstrated her needing to second guess what to do and what to say in an environment that wasn't safe for the person she was supporting. It showed how questions about capacity and choice can complicate practitioners' actions where there is substance use and the need for some of the myths about 'lifestyle' choices and capacity to be countered by accurate legal information (Preston-Shoot and Ward, 2021).

This concern about practice, doing the right thing and prioritising the person's comfort and safety flags the need to consider anxieties among staff. It is about ensuring training is available for people to access and they have support if people present them with challenges they're not used to. Professionals other than palliative and end-of-life care specialists will also need support for conversations about death and dying, particularly if the service structure is one that is traditionally a curative service.

Informal caregivers

Of course, formal services and responses are only part of the picture. Informal caregivers – family and friends – usually hold the majority share of caring duties at home and provide care even in formal care settings. Further, almost a quarter of deaths occur at home (NEoLCIN, 2018), suggesting that family and friends are likely to be providing the majority of care, in addition to the care provided to those who are ultimately admitted to hospital or care homes. Ewing and Grande's (2018) research recommends that carers should be considered both co-workers and clients in their own right within palliative and end-of-life care services. They point out that carers were always considered a key part of palliative and end-of-life

---

Box 13.1 Individual good practice

- Understand and counter the lack of compassion and care that people using substances will expect from services. Be mindful of how this adversely affects their engagement with professionals and services in general.
- Be knowledgeable about the legislation and the myths that suggest capacity and consent stifle practitioner actions to protect and safeguard vulnerable people.
- Be patient, tolerant and resilient in the face of people being evasive and defensive when you offer care – understand that it is not (usually) personal but a normalised survival strategy.
- Consider what their communication needs might be, including their level of health literacy. Do they need a different format of communication?
- Consider whether any non-cooperation may be a lack of understanding of what they're being told, or what they're being asked to do? Do they understand their end-of-life prognosis?
- Be familiar with the language to use and to avoid in relation to substance use and end-of-life care. For example, terms such as alcoholic or addict are full of negative stereotypes and need to be avoided. Terms such as palliative care may not be understood, and people may be frightened by mention of a hospice thinking people just go there to die.
- Develop good individual relationships with people in other agencies – call and ask for help and advice – it opens the door and aids collaborative working.
- Know which local services can support people in terms of their housing, substance use, debt management, immigration status and so on. A quick check on the internet for your local services will help.
- Be prepared to advocate – assertively – for the right of the person to have good quality care and to receive medication appropriate to their condition and tolerance levels.
- Remember the commonality of abuse histories in people using substances – be trauma informed in your approach.
- Help people overcome internalised stigma by demonstrating care and warmth and explicitly countering any pejorative statements they make about themselves.

---

care from the beginning of the movement. They theorise that the absence of, or inconsistency in, carer support relates to them not being 'viewed as true clients of services' (p. 9) and, therefore, a legitimate group for assessment and intervention.

As Wright et al. (Chapter 4) point out, carers require information, knowledge and support from formal services to protect their own health and wellbeing while caring for others to the best of their abilities and taking the strain and costs that would otherwise fall on formal services. They highlight the emotional toll caregiving can take on family and friends which is why there needs to be support and clear communication to maximise appropriate care giving. In her chapter on mental ill health, substance use and end-of-life care, Webb (Chapter 7) highlights the evidence for shared or integrated care that is meant to include informal support systems. However, as she points out, the fragmentation of health and social care services needs to be overcome for the goal of shared and integrated care to be fully realised.

There is, however, an alternate view that needs considering. Family caregivers are not always supportive and can hinder care. Higgs (Chapter 8) points out that people can face stigma and discrimination within the family from adult family members. Wright et al. (Chapter 4) flag the thorny issue of how family and friends can hinder care through their own substance use and related behaviours. This can result in formal care staff needing to find time to plan safe medication dispensing and storage or manage disruptive behaviour in in-patient facilities. Clear policy and practice guidance and supportive family systems are likely to go some way to addressing this behaviour more consistently.

System characteristics

While many of these chapters have called for an increased knowledge and skills base for individual professions and professionals, and an improvement in organisational policy, this is only part of the picture. Attention needs to be paid to the structure of the services and systems within which they operate. It is unsatisfactory to make recommendations for overstretched professionals to learn and do more without addressing the systemic failings much higher up.

However, evidence suggests that full system change to mandate closer working with other agencies and to integrate social and health care has achieved very little. Reed et al. (2021) report on the moves towards integration of social and health care in the four countries of the UK. They reflect that there is a great deal of time spent and expense in restructuring systems that can distract from the main focus:

> No matter how sensible the rationale for organisational restructuring may be, it takes time and headspace to deliver and can divert attention away from the core aim of improving service delivery for people.
>
> (Reed et al., 2021:3)

They point out that new structures are unlikely to lead to improved collaboration and that the real change lies at a relational level rather than a structural one supported by investment in the capacity and skills of their integration partners.

We argue that health and social care services have not been designed to be inclusive of the needs of the more marginalised populations discussed in this text. The delivery of care remains fragmented in spite of aspirations for integrated and shared care (Reed et al, 2021). Health systems are designed to be curative and social care systems are designed to safeguard and support people's wellbeing. There can be a tension between the two approaches leaving the person in the middle trying to navigate their care or absenting themselves from such care because of its complexity.

Individuals, families and professionals seem to agree that holistic services that address a range of the person's needs allow for better care and greater flexibility. The intersectional needs identified in this text cannot be met well by single-focussed services alone. To address this, we propose a new service model that builds upon Brophy and Colclough's (Chapter 9) five broad system characteristics:

1   *Value-driven, personalised care*
2   *A shift in focus to work with uncertainty and enable future planning*
3   *Effective communication*
4   *Education, training and collaboration*
5   *Multi-disciplinary team working.*

The new ComCAS service model (Complex case management and assertive outreach) would sit astride the other services and would seek to embed a consistency of care delivery to people with multiple needs at, or near, the end of their lives. It would not replace the other services, but it would provide an expertise in complex needs and provide a case management function for people whose access to services is currently limited and marginal.

Figure 13.1 identifies the key professions for working with people using substances at the end of their lives but, as this edited collection demonstrates, additional knowledge and expertise may be necessary. Additional specialist roles may be seconded or co-opted to the team as defined by local need.

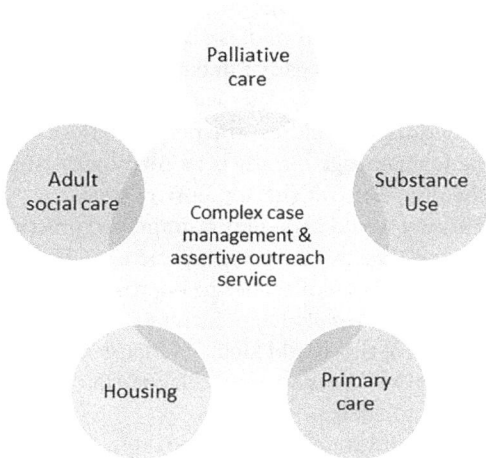

Figure 13.1 ComCAS service model for multiple disadvantage and end-of-life care.

This is not a new model in a wider sense. It is similar in approach to established multi-agency hubs for safeguarding children or tackling sexual violence (Home Office, 2014). It involves a range of professionals developing a new team, ideally co-located, who would also reach back into their own single discipline services in a liaison role to support learning, understanding and collaboration.

The new service would comprise:

- experienced professionals with expertise in multi-agency working and collaboration as well as expertise in two or more complex needs
- a case management approach to ensure consistent and coordinated care for people with multiple needs that works alongside each of the partner agencies
- an assertive outreach component to reach people facing health inequality, and who are currently excluded from services due to a range of barriers
- co-location for ease of communication and shared knowledge
- commitment to information sharing, transparency, developing shared tools and coordinated intervention
- an agreed leadership and management structure
- a commitment to joint training and education within single service teams.

The model does not preclude improved practice at individual and organisational levels and the need to fill policy gaps, but it does identify the additional effort that needs to be taken with people who are not currently accessing care. It also acknowledges the experience and seniority required to coordinate the care of someone whose needs are complex and can be otherwise time consuming for existing services with limited resources. It would go some way to overcoming the environmental and 'situational constraints' of particular disciplinary processes and boundaries identified by Lightfoot and Orford (1986) in their classic article comparing social work and nursing approaches to working with drinkers.

Importantly, the model, with staffing from mixed disciplines and areas of expertise, will overtly demonstrate an understanding of the intersectionality of areas of need and the cumulative negative impact of these experiences in people's lives. The ComCAS team would, together with the person (and family caregivers where appropriate), identify and address the person's priorities while keeping the 'other' experts in the team engaged in the person's progress and care and ready to step forward with their expertise at the appropriate time.

A structure of this kind would also support improved practitioner wellbeing by drawing on others' knowledge in the team, experiencing better service provision, and supporting single discipline colleagues to improve their knowledge and care. Furthermore, it aligns with the global approach to reducing health inequities embedded in the aspirations of the World Health Organisation's (WHO, 1946) constitution through supportive 'cross sector' collaboration to engage communities and support their efforts to address inequities.

Most importantly, it would enable people who often have limited resources and capacity to respond to the demands of multiple agencies and multiple appointments at multiple agencies, to receive the care they deserve at the end of life.

Peacock and Turner (Chapter 12) also concluded that a new model was needed within prisons. Trying to fit older prisoners with complex needs at end of life into the existing 'vulnerable prisoner' (VP) units within prisons was rejected by the prisoners due to the reputation of the VP units for housing sex offenders. Therefore, older people avoided them and were unlikely to get the additional level of care they needed among mainstream prisoners. They called for a new 'older prisoner' unit that could cater for the growing population of older prisoners with complex health and social care needs.

Similarly, in her chapter on mental health, substance use and end-of-life care, Webb (Chapter 7) calls for a move towards a person-centred recovery approach that targets quality of life rather than symptom control as the 'gateway' to palliative thinking (Strand et al., 2020) – an approach that a ComCAS model could adopt. Developing a service such as ComCAS would avoid what Higgs (Chapter 8) refers to in his Australia-focussed chapter, as the constant negotiation with service providers just to get appropriate care. It would also recognise that, in supporting people who are marginalised, motivation to engage with care and care providers is co-created between practitioner and the person with experience (Mahmood, 2021). Access and engagement are more likely to happen with practitioners who are committed to supporting someone with complex needs at the end of life and who offers a non-judgemental approach.

Conclusion

Fundamental to the lives and experiences reflected in this book is the issue of social and professional attitudes and values towards people with multiple and intersectional needs at, or near, the end of their lives. Despite calls for the correction of health inequalities at the end of life, backed by equality legislation, evidence suggests there has been little movement, thus sustaining an unequal and unjust system of care that for many people lacks dignity and comfort at the end of their lives.

Peacock and Turner (Chapter 12) ask what is 'just', for whom and who decides, when it comes to end-of-life care. Does a person in prison with cancer and substance problems deserve the same care as someone in the community with substance problems? Such questions give us pause. It makes us reflect sharply on which groups of people or characteristics we consider less deserving than others and challenges us to ensure our own and others' prejudices do not get in the way of compassionate care for people at, or near, the end of their lives. For some people discussed in this book, discrimination and prejudice are based on inherent characteristics such as ethnicity or learning disabilities. For others, it is about acquired behaviours such as substance use, offending or prostitution – behaviours that are erroneously considered 'lifestyle choices', as if anyone would choose the approbation and judgement those behaviours so often bring.

While action at individual and organisational levels is necessary to maximise health equalities, we need to adopt a multi-pronged approach. We need to recognise that endless demands on poorly resourced health and social care professionals and agencies to know more and do better with people with complex intersecting needs will only achieve minimal change. We need to make a more concerted effort to share good practice far and wide and ultimately this is the goal of this text. We need to change direction and add to our existing services an approach that will compliment and support existing services while offering a holistic and person-centred approach to caring for people using substances at the end of their lives. A service based on acceptance, harm minimisation, dignity and respect.

References

Care Quality Commission. (2016) *A different ending: addressing inequalities in end of life care*. CQC CQC–317–052016. Available online at: https://www.cqc.org.uk/sites/default/files/20160505%20CQC_EOLC_OVERVIEW_FINAL_3.pdf [Accessed 29th March 2022].

Decorte, I., Verfaillie, F., Moureau, L., Meynendonckx, S., Van Ballaer, K., De Geest, I. and Liégeois, A. (2020) Oyster care: An innovative palliative approach towards SPMI patients. *Frontiers in Psychiatry*, 11. Available online at: https://www.frontiersin.org/article/10.3389/fpsyt.2020.00509 DOI=10.3389/fpsyt.2020.00509.

Ewing, G. and Grande, G. (2018) *Providing comprehensive, person-centred assessment and support for family carers towards the end of life: 10 recommendations for achieving organisational change*. London: Hospice UK, 2018. Available online at: carers-report---10-recommendations-for-achieving-organisational-change_final.pdf (hospiceuk.org) [Accessed 21st March 2022].

Galvani, S. and Wright, S. (2019) *Supporting people with substance problems at the end of life. Palliative and end of life care for people with alcohol and drug problems* (Policy Standards). Manchester: Manchester Metropolitan University. Available online at: https://endoflifecaresubstanceuse.com/wp-content/uploads/2022/02/Policy-Standards-SU-and-EoLC-May-2019.pdf [Accessed 4th March 2022].

Galvani, S., Wright, S. and Witham, G. (2019) *Supporting people with substance problems at end of life (Good Practice Guidance)*. Manchester: Manchester Metropolitan University. Available online at: https://endoflifecaresubstanceuse.com/wp-content/uploads/2022/02/Good-practice-guidance-EoLC-and-SU-April-2019-Web-version.pdf [Accessed 4th March 2022].

Home Office. (2014) *Multi agency working and information sharing project final report*. Available online at: https://assets.publishing.service.gov.uk/government/uploads/system/uploads/attachment_data/file/338875/MASH.pdf [Accessed 15th March 2022].

Lightfoot, P. J. C. and Orford, J. (1986) Helping agents' attitudes towards alcohol-related problems: situations vacant? A test and elaboration of a model. *British Journal of Addiction*, 81, 749–756. DOI: 10.1111/j.1360-0443.1986.tb00402.x

Mahmood, F. (2021) 'Exploring reasons for clients' non-attendance at appointments within a community-based alcohol service: clients' and practitioners' perspectives.' PhD thesis. Manchester Metropolitan University. FaisalMahmood_14501562_PhDThesis_Final.pdf (mmu.ac.uk) [Accessed 28th March 2022].

National End of Life Care Intelligence Network (NEoLCIN). (2018) *Atlas of variation for palliative and end of life care in England. Reducing unwarranted variation to improve health outcomes and value*. London: Public Health England. Available online at: https://fingertips.phe.org.uk/documents/Atlas%20of%20variation%20for%20palliative%20and%20end%20of%20life%20care%20Final.pdf [Accessed 4th March 2022].

National Palliative and End of Life Care Partnership. (2021) *Ambitions for palliative and end of life care: a national framework for local action 2021–2026.* Available online at: https://www.england.nhs.uk/blog/renewing-our-ambitions-for-palliative-and-end-of-life-care/ [Accessed 2nd August 2021].

National Palliative and End of Life Care Partnership (NPELCP). (2015) *Ambitions for palliative and end of life care: a national framework for local action 2015–2020.* https://www.nationalvoices.org.uk/sites/default/files/public/publications/ambitions-for-palliative-and-end-of-life-care.pdf

OHID. (2022) *Local alcohol profiles for England – Hospital admissions due to alcohol.* Available online at: https://fingertips.phe.org.uk/profile/local-alcohol-profiles/supporting-information/Admissions2

ONS. (2021a) *Deaths related to drug poisoning in England and Wales from 1993 to 2020, by cause of death, sex, age and substances involved in the death.* Available online at: file:///C:/Users/55123422/Downloads/Deaths%20related%20to%20drug%20poisoning%20in%20England%20and%20Wales%202020%20registrations.pdf [accessed 4th March 2022]

ONS. (2021b) *Alcohol-specific deaths in the UK: registered in 2020.* Available online at: https://www.ons.gov.uk/peoplepopulationandcommunity/healthandsocialcare/causesofdeath/bulletins/alcoholrelateddeathsintheunitedkingdom/registeredin2020#:~:text=1.-,Main%20points, time%20series%20began%20in%202001. [Accessed 4th March 2022].

Payne, S., Hughes, S., Wilkinson, J., Hasselaar, J. and Preston, N. (2019) Recommendations on priorities for integrated palliative care: transparent expert consultation with international leaders for the InSuP-C project. *BMC Palliative Care*, 18, 32. https://doi.org/10.1186/s12904-019-0418-5 Recommendations on priorities for integrated palliative care: transparent expert consultation with international leaders for the InSuP-C project | BMC Palliative Care | Full Text (biomedcentral.com) [accessed 3 May 2022]

Preston-Shoot, M. and Ward, M. (2021) *How to use legal powers to safeguard highly vulnerable dependent drinkers in England and Wales.* London: Alcohol Change UK. Available online at: https://alcoholchange.org.uk/publication/how-to-use-legal-powers-to-safeguard-highly-vulnerable-dependent-drinkers [Accessed 4th March 2022].

Reed, S., Oung. C., Davies, J., Dayan, M. and Scobie, S. (2021) *Integrating health and social care: A comparison of policy and progress across the four countries of the UK.* Research report, Nuffield Trust. Available online at: https://www.nuffieldtrust.org.uk/research/-integrating-health-and-social-care-a-comparison-of-policy-and-progress-across-the-four-countries-of-the-uk#report-overview [Accessed 4th March 2022].

Roscoe, S., Pryce, R., Buykx, P., Gavens, L. and Meier, P.S. (2022), Is disinvestment from alcohol and drug treatment services associated with treatment access, completions and related harm? An analysis of English expenditure and outcomes data. *Drug and Alcohol Review*, 41, 54–61. DOI: 10.1111/dar.13307

Strand, M., Sjostrand, M. and Lindblad, A. (2020) A palliative care approach in psychiatry: Clinical implications. *BMC Medical Ethics*, 21, 29. DOI: 10.1186/s12910-020-00472-8

World Health Organization. (1946) *Constitution of the World Health Organization.* Basic Documents, Geneva: World Health Organization.

World Health Organization. (2020) 'Palliative Care.' Palliative care (who.int) [Accessed 3rd May 2022].

Index

Note: **Bold** page numbers refer to tables; *italic* page numbers refer to figures and page numbers followed by "n" denote endnotes.

For Product Safety Concerns and Information please contact our EU
representative GPSR@taylorandfrancis.com
Taylor & Francis Verlag GmbH, Kaufingerstraße 24, 80331 München, Germany